School-Based Multisystemic
Interventions for Mass Trauma

School-Based Multisystemic Interventions for Mass Trauma

Avigdor Klingman
Faculty of Education
University of Haifa, Israel

and

Esther Cohen
School of Education
The Hebrew University of Jerusalem, Israel

Kluwer Academic/Plenum Publishers
New York   Boston   Dortrecht   London   Moscow

Library of Congress Cataloging-in-Publication Data

Klingman, Avigdor.
  School-based multisystemic interventions for mass trauma / by Avigdor Klingman and Esther Cohen
    p. cm.
  Includes bibliographical references and index.
  ISBN 0-306-48066-2
  1. Post-traumatic disorder in children—Prevention. 2. Psychic trauma in children—Prevention. 3. School children—Mental health services. 4. Child disaster victims—Mental health services. I. Cohen, Esther, Ph. D. II. Title.

RJ056.P55K56 2004
618.92'85210651–dc22   2003060445

IBSN: 0-306-48066-2

© 2004 Kluwer Academic/Plenum Publishers
233 Spring Street, New York, New York 10013

http://www.wkap.nl/

10   9   8   7   6   5   4   3   2   1

A C.I.P. record for this book is available from the Library of Congress

Permission for books published in Europe: permissions@wkap.nl
Permission for books published in the United States of America: permissions@wkap.com

Printed in the United States of America

Foreword

Since Sept 11, 2001 and the events that have followed, namely the anthrax scare, the Washington sniper, and the continual terrorist bombings in various parts of the world, it has become clear that society and its agencies need to be prepared for disaster. Schools, in particular, where children spend hours of their time, need to think through ways to become prepared for disaster. This volume has as its intention to provide an understanding of mass trauma and its impact on school systems, and to present a plan for school systems to put in place in preparation for such eventualities. It is a volume that presents both a scientific and theoretical framework as well as hands on techniques that school administrators and mental health professionals can put into place.

Who better to present this material than these two authors, both of whom have experience dealing with disaster both in Israel and in the United States? Avigdor Klingman is Professor in the Counseling and Therapy Division of the Faculty of Education of the University of Haifa and has served as Head of the State Disaster Crises Intervention Division of the Psychological Services of the Ministry of Education in Israel. His work has been selected by the American Psychological Association's Division of Child, Youth, and Family as a model program for service delivery. His work includes research on children's and adolescents' stress reactions and coping in war and warlike situations and the study of the effects of school-based primary prevention and stress inoculation programs. Esther Cohen is Chair of the Graduate Program for Educational and Child-Clinical Psychology at the Hebrew University in Jerusalem. She has been engaged in clinical work with children, families, and groups affected by war and terrorism, served as the head of the preschool psychological services for the city of Jerusalem and in the aftermath of 9/11 lectured, trained, and consulted at the Ackerman Institute, the NYU Child Study Center, and the NYU International Trauma Studies Center. Each of these authors brings a unique and powerful perspective to the material.

The book is divided into two parts: the theoretical and empirical background and then the multisystemic intervention programs for schools. Each of these parts is further divided into pertinent sections. The authors have succeeded in making a clear and understandable presentation of the material in a way that can be useful to academics and trainers as well as school personnel who have to make decisions and plans.

This book will serve both as a reference tool and as a toolkit. It is comprehensive without being pedantic and detailed enough without being disrespectful to the reader. The suggested interventions range from preventive to therapeutic and from classroom-based and teacher led, to professional mental health.

The examples of clinical interventions are compelling and elucidating. There is particular focus on bringing all of the players in the schools into the planning loop and in making sure that parents are involved. While this may seem to be obvious, it is something often forgotten in our work in the schools. It is clear that if all of the players are not called upon to participate both in the planning and in the execution of the plan, it will not work. Mental health personnel should certainly be in the foreground and in the leadership when it comes to the kinds of programs that need to be developed. But that will depend on how the particular school is structured and how accessible the mental health personnel make themselves. Teachers have to be considered and trained while dealt with respectfully. Clearly, the culture of the school has to be taken into account and the culture of the children has to be taken into account. Where there is a disconnection between the school and the family, the program will not work. But that is true for the entire educational program. An additional focus is placed on positive coping, resilience, and the role of the mental health professional in enhancing these processes in schools.

It is unfortunate that the events of the last two years have led to the pressing need for this book. In my own work in schools post 9/11, it became painfully clear to me how unprepared our schools were to deal with the massive needs of children, teachers, and parents in the wake of the World Trade Center attack. Although it is probably true that a system can never be prepared enough and that disasters will continue to surprise and overwhelm, this book will serve as a blueprint for thinking about and planning for responses to disaster.

We need to be thankful that this book will help us acquire an attitude of preparedness and a way to develop and execute appropriate plans.

LAURA BARBANEL, Ed.D., ABPP
Professor Emerita
Brooklyn College, City University of New York

Preface

Extending more than three decades, our involvement in the lives of Israeli children and adults affected by mass-trauma events related to war and terrorism has spanned a gamut of professional roles as: school mental health staff, clinicians, consultants, trainers, university teachers, and researchers. While A.K. has already received recognition by the American Psychological Association for his school-based model, we came to realize the full extent of our cumulative expertise in the aftermath of the terrorist attacks of September 11, 2001 in the United States. E.C., who happened to be on sabbatical in New York City during that year, became a participant-observer in numerous professional activities initiated in response to the trauma. This helped sharpen the relevance of our experiences for those heretofore unacquainted with the challenges presented by mass trauma of this magnitude, especially mental health professionals and agencies that work in the school system, or are associated with it, as well as educational leadership and school administration. In this book, we attempt to provide first a systematic review of the theory and findings relevant to mass disasters, their impact on children, and postdisaster stress processing and positive coping. Second, we try to establish a conceptual basis for schoolwide preventive interventions. Third, we present a comprehensive multisystemic intervention plan involving schoolchildren, parents, school personnel, and community agencies.

The ability of the survivors with whom we have worked to create meaningful lives, in spite of adversity, inspired the endeavor undertaken in this book.

AVIGDOR KLINGMAN
ESTHER COHEN

Acknowledgments

I n bringing this book to fruition, many individuals over numerous years were involved – in our thought processes, in our conceptualizations, and in our experiences in the school systems in Israel and the United States. We extend our thanks to all those who shared with us their trepidations and trauma on the one hand, and their expertise and advise on the other. Without a doubt, this book stemmed from their yearnings and entreating demands for a comprehensive intervention model that could attempt to soften the blow of disaster on the entire school community.

I, A.K., would like to thank my wife, Ayala, for the utmost support she gave me while I spent long hours conducting, supervising, and following up on mass trauma crisis interventions, and my son Opher and my daughter Leat who, while growing up, were unwitting partners to my involvement in these interventions.

I, E.C., am grateful to my colleagues at the NYU Child Study Center, and at the Ackerman Institute for the Family, who provided a most enriching, dialectical, and supportive environment in New York City, during my sabbatical year that began just prior to the events of September 2001, and instigated my involvement with this book. It was, however, the constant encouragement of my husband Akiba, and the joy that my children Orlee and Amitai, and especially my grandchildren Eli and Carmel, have brought to my life, that made this effort possible.

Finally, our editor, Dee B. Ankonina, was invaluable in challenging and organizing our thinking and putting the final manuscript together.

Contents

Part **I**

Theoretical and Empirical Background on Mass Disasters, Stress Responses, and Positive Responding

Section A

Introduction: Triggers and Assumptions

The outlook presented in this book on ways of helping children cope with mass disasters is grounded in a critical consideration of presently emerging needs, and lessons from actual traumatic experiences and interventions. This outlook also reflects a choice of perspective, which values school-based, multisystemic, preventive interventions, a choice justified by supporting theory and research, and articulated in our underlying assumptions. The following chapters on the events triggering this book and our preliminary assumptions are designed to introduce the reader to our theoretical, conceptual, and professional outlook, which will be detailed later.

Chapter 1

The Events Triggering This Book

The writing of this book was spurred by the dramatic escalation in brutal terrorism toward the start of the third millennium, and especially the catastrophic events of September 11, 2001 in the United States, as well as the relentless wave of suicide bombers in Israel during the ensuing period. The urgent need to address the psychological aftermath of these events and to ensure better preparation for any future eventuality has become of paramount importance. Naturally, many of the issues discussed in this book were written with these events in mind. The scope of this book, however, is not limited to dealing with school-based responses to the aforementioned or similar acts of terror, but rather aims to tackle a wider spectrum of traumatic experiences.

Civilization has always been under the threat of natural forces and their devastating impact, yet the world today faces even more ominous disasters related to "advanced" technologies. Modern disasters may result from lethal human error, ranging from transportation accidents to biological and chemical industrial accidents, to nuclear reactor failures like in Chernobyl. Perhaps even more difficult to accept are intentional human acts such as the nerve gas infiltration into Tokyo's subway and the anthrax-infected mail in the United States. Moreover, the epidemic-like increase in political and ethnic violence around the world that followed the end of the cold war is resulting in "mass trauma" experienced by millions of civilians, including an escalating number of children (Wright, Masten, & Hubbard, 1997).

WORLDWIDE ESCALATING VIOLENCE

Children the world over are now being exposed, more than ever, to the escalating brutality of war, political violence, ethnic strife, large-scale terrorism, and community and school violence. This rise may be explained by the increase in the incidence of civilian involvement in recent conflicts. Indeed, most contemporary conflicts are not fought between states or armies, nor are they limited to the front lines, thus defying the traditional distinction between combatants and non-combatants. In fact, children, youth, and women become specific targets for violence in some areas of the world (e.g., the Balkans, formerly Yugoslavia). Various conflict zones exploit children for ideological propaganda or enlist them into civil strife activities such as rock throwing at troops or even combat fighting (as in Southeast Asia, Northern Ireland, and the West Bank).

Increased violence impacts the lives of children not only in lands entangled in religious, ethnic, and political strife. Even in the most politically stable, peaceful, and affluent democracies of the world, children face violence that may be described as having reached epidemic proportions (Osofsky & Scheeringa, 1997). One such example was the succession of repeated sniper killings in the Washington DC area over several weeks during October 2002. These shootings, which randomly victimized adults near shopping centers and other public places, including a child near his school, virtually shut down social and community events and lead to massive avoidance of school attendance. Violence in schools is especially disturbing. A 1996 poll conducted in the USA revealed that 47 percent of all teens believed their schools were becoming more violent, and 10 percent feared being shot or hurt by classmates carrying weapons to school (National Center for Educational Statistics, 1998). Even children who are spared the direct experiences of violence or disasters are nevertheless often extensively exposed to them through the media, and thus may be vicariously affected.

A CASE IN POINT: SEPTEMBER 11, 2001

The recent simultaneous terrorist attacks on the World Trade Center (WTC) and Pentagon on September 11, 2001 – which constituted a traumatic event of unprecedented magnitude in the history of the USA – vividly illustrate the effects of collective disaster on children, schools, mental health services, and the community, as well as the new challenges facing these systems. The 9/11 events involved the loss of thousands of civilian lives and enormous destruction to property as well as serious harm to the economy. The attacks rendered an acute impact on the daily lives and psychological well being of New York City's population and generated a wider, rippling impact, for example on the outlying areas around the city, in the Washington DC metropolitan area, and around urban centers in the USA. Many residents of western democracies the world over were engaged in compulsive media watching. According to an epidemiological study conducted 5–8 weeks later, an estimated 7.5% of adults in New York

City, and 20% of those residing in the vicinity of the WTC, were suffering from posttraumatic stress disorder (PTSD) symptomatology. An even higher incidence of recent adult depression emerged (Galea et al., 2002).

Likewise, the 9/11 events confronted children with grave experiences. Some children personally witnessed the horrifying sights of planes flying into buildings, bodies falling, and buildings collapsing. Many children lost a family member and had to deal with grief made more complicated by the traumatic nature of these deaths. Others knew children who were orphaned. An estimated 15,000 children were evacuated from schools, experienced a delayed reunion with their families, and had to adjust to the dislocation of their home or school. And the vast majority of children experienced repeated exposure to vivid graphic televised broadcasts of the atrocity of these attacks and the ensuing terrorism threats, including the anthrax scare.

The results of an epidemiological study conducted six months after the attack afforded an assessment of the event's effects on the mental health of children in the city, beyond the initial acute period. A broad range of mental health difficulties was observed at a higher than expected prevalence among New York City public school children in grades 4–12, especially depression and anxiety (about 10%). Additionally, an estimated 10.5 percent of these schoolchildren (that is, as many as 75,000 children) exhibited symptoms consistent with a PTSD diagnosis (NYC Board of Education website, May 2002; Hoven et. al., 2002). These problems continued to affect the daily functioning of some of the children over the long term, presenting a challenge to their parents and schools.

School personnel, parents, mental health services, and professionals in affected areas, all acutely experienced a lack of preparedness during the 9/11 disaster. Although schools across the board were clearly aware of their obligation to help children return home safely at the time of the disaster, the schools' additional duties were blurred and indefinite with regard to the processing of the trauma. A wide range of responses emerged in handling the unusual circumstances, mainly because, prior to the event, teachers and school administrators had rarely addressed questions related to students' direct or indirect exposure to such tragic events. Many teachers succeeded in overcoming their own confusion and anxiety and in providing their students with necessary information, without overwhelming them. Various schools improvised means to help children feel protected and supported. However, not all schools coped optimally. Anxiety and a wish to overprotect the children motivated some teachers to invent fictitious excuses when explaining to students the need for immediate evacuation of classrooms (e.g., the need to disinfect the building, an overly warm temperature). These fabrications may have caused a loss in teacher credibility during a highly significant moment. A number of teachers found it easier to frame the occurrence as an accident, making it difficult later on to retract this version. A few teachers did not grasp the enormity of the disaster and may have overexposed their students to the event (e.g., going up with the students to the roof of the school building to observe the collapse of the WTC).

In the ensuing weeks, many teachers and school administrators remained confused and unsure about their responsibility for and ability to handle students' psychological reactions to the event. Many felt conflicted about the dilemma of leaving the traumatic event alone or processing it, and unsure about their ability to integrate their "traditional teaching role" with a new, more "therapeutic" role. Some schools managed to enlist additional resources such as extra staff, parents, volunteers, and mental health consultants. In all likelihood, these resources were conducive not only to better monitoring of the overall psychological reactions of the school community, but also to better processing of the trauma through the use of various initiatives and activities, including discussion groups and expressive arts projects.

Compelling new circumstances created by the trauma dictated the agenda in a number of schools. Such circumstances included organizational problems related to dislocation, parental and staff anxieties about health hazards upon returning to the original school site, dealing with the specific problems of children whose families suffered great direct losses, and mounting tensions between ethnic groups. Within the multidisciplinary educational system, it was not always clear who was best equipped to support the schools' decision making processes and efforts to address the unusual challenges, nor how to best coordinate the inputs of administration and policy makers, regional crisis teams, school personnel, independent consultants and agencies, parents, and volunteers.

During the months following the disaster, many schools returned rather quickly to "business as usual," assuming that the distance from the disaster site had protected their students. However, the extent to which children remained psychologically affected by the event, and the need for additional resources, began to be recognized. This led to collaborative professional initiatives, such as those undertaken by the newly formed organization named: The Children's Mental Health Alliance (http;// www.cmha.org).

LESSONS LEARNED

In looking back at the handling of the crisis and its aftermath by the various relevant institutions and organizations, we commend their good will, devotion, and capacity for improvisation, but clearly these qualities do not suffice in handling a tragedy of such magnitude. This holds equally true for mental health agencies and professionals. Many mental health agencies and professionals felt anxious and ill prepared for dealing with such a crisis. For instance, some agencies opened walk-in clinics only to discover that the service was of little use at the time following the event, as families seemed to need to remain close to home and to concentrate on the pressing task of reorganizing their lives. In the schools, it became apparent to mental health professionals and administrators that psychologists' and school counselors' traditional training had not adequately prepared them for mass emergencies. What is more, the wide-ranging scope of the required interventions demonstrated that no single school or system possessed sufficient professional resources to provide those services needed to cope with such an enormous disaster. Various leading institutions and mental health agencies responded rapidly to the emergent needs by disseminating mental health information through the Internet and by conducting open seminars about expected reactions and recommended coping strategies. However, as professionals in the aftermath of the disaster began calling for new assessment procedures and treatment models, the lack of clear professional consensus emerged regarding how to conceptualize, organize, deliver, and evaluate those services.

The future role of child mental health professionals in preparing for and participating in the management of similar possible events remains contentious. Much debatable detail remains to be worked out in the organizational and professional spheres: Who should continue to support the children, the school organization, the school staff, and the families over the long term in the processing of the trauma? Who is best equipped to follow up on and help students in need? What are the best practices for these interventions? These questions pertain to a broad range of disciplines: school personnel and administration, policy makers at various levels, and mental health professionals involved in children's care systems.

Lessons must be drawn to improve the future functioning of institutions, systems, and individuals in order to minimize casualties and to prevent physical and psychological damage. In this book, we hope to contribute to this enterprise by focusing on ways to protect children's mental health via the most significant systems in their lives: family, school, and mental health and other community services.

OUR BOOK

To elucidate the best intervention practices, we will draw both on theory and research, as well as from our experience both through preventive interventions in the school system and through clinical practice. Although recommendations based on empirical research data are most valuable, research in the area of trauma response is limited and problematic, given the complex and unique conditions and the various operational pressures involved in each disaster.

To address these limitations, we will propose that situation-specific interventions be creatively tailored on the basis of principles drawn both from research and from prior experiences in crisis intervention. We attribute great value to the extensive experience accumulated by professionals involved in crisis interventions around the world and especially in trauma-stricken areas, even if this experience is not accompanied by clear research evidence. Such professional experiences may include case material, anecdotes, media reports, professional observations, as well as accounts of interventions with schoolchildren following large-scale disasters by our colleagues in Israel (e.g., Klingman, Raviv, & Stein, 2000) and elsewhere. If examined in light of existing theorizing and research, these accounts may become a source for defining and refining principles, guidelines, and practical recommendations for future practice.

This book is not intended to be a concrete, step-by-step "how-to" manual. We do offer specific suggestions, examples, and field-tested illustrations within an organizational framework. However, our major objectives consist of constructing a framework for conceptualizing issues; deepening the understanding of the dynamics involved in children's coping with disaster and trauma at the personal, interpersonal, systemic, and inter-systemic levels; and proposing a working model for intervention that is based on an explicated rationale and guiding principles. It is our hope that this endeavor will assist those agencies and individuals who hold responsibility for the welfare of children to proactively generate, adapt, tailor, modify, and carry out plans to meet children's needs at various stages of each potentially traumatic event as it unfolds.

Chapter 2

Our Preliminary Assumptions

We will now present some of the core assumptions underlying the approach of this book. Our approach places an emphasis on predisaster preparedness via school-based multisystemic activities that will enhance children's coping and adjustment in the event of a disaster. Further, this approach focuses on school personnel and families, both to foster their own resilience and adaptation, and to empower them to carry out a variety of ongoing and dynamic preventive and therapeutic interventions, when and after disaster strikes, designed to enhance recovery via the natural support systems. The exposition of our ten core assumptions, next, can serve as a rationale and an introduction to our mindset concerning the school-based multisystemic preventive approach to disaster.

The *first assumption* underlying the school-based multisystemic approach asserts that humans possess strong mechanisms for **natural recovery** from potentially traumatic events. Consequently, intervention efforts must be cognizant of these mechanisms and capitalize on them. Human recovery includes the ability to regain a sense of efficacy through activity, to affiliate with others in times of need, and to solve problems creatively in times of duress. Additional recovery mechanisms comprise the ability to process emotions through the use of symbolic and expressive means, to create new narratives out of experiences and to be inspired by their meanings, and to employ many other human talents and resources in coping with disaster. Intervention planning must create the conditions that activate, channel, and support these human capacities.

Our *second assumption* asserts that **preparation is essential for better coping**. A mass disaster threatens and challenges habitual modes of individual and organizational coping. When disaster strikes, individuals often feel confused, paralyzed, and overwhelmed by the unfamiliar challenges; organizations often become overburdened with urgent unfamiliar tasks and function chaotically. Yet preplanning is not a simple endeavor, considering the already overburdening workload of school personnel, the remoteness of mass disaster, and the uneasiness that this possibility arouses. Overstrained schools and reluctant staff may contribute to the avoidance of such preparatory efforts.

Nevertheless, we believe that it is the responsibility of any organization, and especially those involved in the welfare of children, like schools, to take steps toward preparing for future hazards. Our experience during various disasters in Israel and the USA strongly indicates that schools can become a central change agent in the lives of children and their families, can be instrumental in building children's resilience, and can successfully alleviate distress (and possibly physical casualties and the risks of PTSD) following disasters. Relying on organizations' and individuals' spontaneous resourcefulness in managing unfamiliar events, when mass disaster strikes, is risky and ineffective. Common sense dictates that an atmosphere of relative calmness prior to traumatic events can favorably encourage organizing, thinking ahead, and problem solving.

An additional rationale supporting the merit of investing in school preparedness for disaster comprises the meaningful secondary benefits of such a crisis plan to schools' ordinary everyday operation, and not only when disaster occurs. Such an investment can improve individual and systemic coping with mundane, less severe problems and can foster a more supportive, collaborative, proactive, and responsible school climate. These benefits should be strongly underscored when offering the option of disaster preparedness to schools.

The *third assumption* concerns the key role played by **significant familial attachment figures** in helping children cope and adjust. Significant adults who cope effectively and regulate their own emotions during stressful times can become more attuned to children's needs. Children rely on adults in their natural environment for emotional as well as for physical survival. They need protection from both external and internal threats to their safety, self-esteem, resiliency, and sense of well-being. Most families intuitively rush to protect their children from physical harm but may find the task of preventing emotional injury far more challenging. It is the family, and especially the parents, who can provide the child with a psychological "safe space" and whose support should comprise a major arena for intervention in disaster (Norris et al., 2002a, 2002b).

The *fourth assumption* claims that, in addition to the family, the **school can and should be viewed as a natural support system**. In times of mass crisis, to support children in dealing with new stresses and in processing unusual events, the adaptation of preexisting familiar support networks such as schools far outweighs the benefits of creating new frameworks. The school constitutes children's natural community system, where they spend most of their waking hours, socialize with peers, and learn to benefit from adult knowledge. Following disaster, the school offers a central community meeting place for diverse adults, which exposes students to a

network of supportive figures: parents, classroom teachers, school counselors, the school nurse, administrative and support staff, school or visiting
psychologists, social workers, other community professionals, etc.

Familiar, caring school faculty and accepting classmates play a crucial
role in enabling the child to experience and integrate complex realities in
a psychologically safe environment. The school's classroom, small group,
and individual interventions may contribute greatly to the potential for
prevention, healthy coping enhancement, and wellness optimization after
a traumatic event. This potential role for school staff requires a diversion
from the traditional teaching role, and in some cases may be met with
individual and organizational resistance due to personnel's own anxieties,
sense of insecurity in handling such tasks, and lack of adequate preparedness. Adherence to the habitual teaching role in the aftermath of disaster is
greatly compromised due to students' preoccupation with trauma-related
contents and difficulties concentrating and regulating their emotional reactions. In-service teacher training can focus on ways to adopt new skills
and adapt existing skills to meet students' needs at unusual times. Such
training will certainly serve teachers well in coping with extraordinary
instances of mass disaster but also can contribute significantly to teachers'
professional development in handling everyday student crises.

The *fifth assumption* upholds the **greater impact of multisystemic interventions**. We purport that coordinated interventions, enacted simultaneously in more than one relevant system, will render a much stronger
impact in producing change than will the cumulative impact of separate
interventions. The benefits inherent in adopting a systemic rather than
individual approach in dealing with children's problems received much
theoretical and empirical support in the last decade (Mash & Barkley,
1998). In particular, the systemic approach evidenced intervention efficacy
and preventive benefits. When dealing with especially difficult problems,
the systemic approach has recently been widened to include multisystemic
interventions (Henggeler, Schenwald, Bordin, Rowland, & Cunningham,
1998). The thinking behind these programs, based both on systems
theory (e.g., Bateson, 1972; Minuchin, 1985) and on social ecology
(Bronfenbrenner, 1979), holds that assessment and intervention should be
conducted within the natural ecology of the youth and family (e.g., home,
school, and community). Collection of information from multiple sources
like the child, parents, siblings, peers, and teachers is expected to maximize
ecological validity and to facilitate intervention design. Multisystem interventions target key factors within and between the multiple systems in
which the child is embedded. This recent development has proven particularly effective in treating intractable, pervasive community problems
such as antisocial behavior problems in youth (Henggeler et al., 1998) and
substance abuse (Landau et al., 2000). The multisystemic approach seems
especially relevant for mass disaster situations, in which intense emotional
experiences are shared by victims, witnesses, significant others in their

lives, other adults, and the mental health professionals. Thus, coordinated intervention should simultaneously incorporate those various systems in the students' environment – the family, education system, and community – that should be most effective in promoting children's successful processing of and coping with the potentially traumatic experience.

The *sixth assumption* argues that intervention for individual children and related adults should be offered in *the least stigmatizing context of treatment*. This principle corresponds to the legal requirement that children with special needs should receive services in the least restrictive educational environment possible. The obvious rationale for this principle is to prevent added harmful effects due to the affected individual's anxiety, confusion, or shame regarding the legitimacy of his or her unusual reactions to the adverse situation. Researchers have unanimously advocated the normalization of a wide range of responses and coping mechanisms, not only in words but also in determining the settings for therapeutic intervention. Interventions carried out in natural group settings such as the classroom, after school program, school assembly, staff room, and parent group are less stigmatizing than interventions conducted for selected individuals in settings such as hospitals and mental health agencies. The school setting's atmosphere of shared trauma and its group interventions' lower stigma level highlight schools as a preferred location for effective child intervention, especially for school-based group interventions (Chemtob, Nakashima, & Carlson, 2002; Saltzman, Steinberg, Layne, Aisenberg, & Pynoos, 2002).

The *seventh assumption* proposes that *prevention comprises the best immediate community response* to a potentially traumatic event. Current research demonstrates that children who were exposed to stressful and traumatic events are at risk for a variety of future emotional, behavioral, and physical difficulties (van der Kolk, McFarlane, & Weiseth, 1996). Prevention offers a proactive approach designed to counteract the possible effects associated with exposure to disaster. Generally, preventive efforts must be directed toward identifying mechanisms relevant to bolstering compensatory factors and decreasing the probability of maladaptation (in individuals as well as in organizations). Primary preventive actions at different phases (before, during, and after disaster) should strengthen children's existing support networks by providing guidance and training to school personnel and by planning policies and procedures that aim to build children's resiliency and prevent further psychological damage. Such preventive activities may include the development of a crisis response plan and standard operating procedures, predesignation of a school crisis team, rapid resumption of routine after disaster to ensure continuity, teacher-mediated classroom crisis interventions, curricular modifications, adaptations in personnel's roles, expressive arts activities to promote emotional processing and interpersonal communication, and more.

The *eighth assumption* maintains that schools can function as postdisaster intervention sites not only for school-wide preventative initiatives targeting the whole student population, but also for more *specialized school-based interventions and long-term follow-up programs targeting those at risk or those who already have developed chronic maladaptive symptomatology*. To achieve long-term stabilization and healing, schools may require support, training, and ongoing collaborative ties with professional mental health agencies. Schools boast the capacity to monitor students' responses systematically on a daily basis via intensive staff contact with the children. This capacity affords schools a unique role as the basis for ongoing screening and identification of children's intervention needs, as well as for follow-up information regarding the effect of various therapeutic interventions. Long-term intervention includes continued processing of the trauma, minimization of its residual effects, and dealing with its repeated reminders in the school's everyday functioning. Additionally, it involves the systematic identification and referral of new (delayed onset) cases of posttraumatic reactions, follow-up of previously identified students, and appropriate reintegration of convalescing students who were physically and/or psychologically affected and are returning to regular school activities after receiving treatment.

The *ninth assumption* upholds that **an emphasis on wellness optimization in trauma work is preferable to an emphasis on the reduction of posttraumatic symptomatology**. Much of the current emphasis in the trauma literature, especially in cognitive behavioral models, lies on targeting and reducing PTSD symptomatology. In contrast, we emphasize the *salutogenic approach* (Antonovsky, 1987, 1990) and ideas from the literature on trauma-induced growth (Calhoun & Tedeschi, 1999) to promote health in trauma work. Disasters, like any crisis, can mobilize previously untapped potentials, empower individuals through a stronger sense of coherence, and create an enhanced climate of community belonging, thus reducing survivors' feelings of powerlessness. Moreover, the struggle with a traumatic event may lead to positive gains such as strengthened relationships with others, increased intimacy and closeness, altruistic activities, an augmented experience of oneself as capable and self-reliant, and a greater and richer appreciation of life.

The *tenth and last assumption* suggests that **clinical and preventive approaches should complement one another**. Two major, seemingly contradictory trends characterize the recent literature on trauma intervention: the "clinical" approach influenced by the medical model, and the "psychosocial" or "psychoeducational" approach influenced by community psychology, the field of prevention, and positive psychology. These two trends reflect the two dominant treatment approaches in the field of childhood trauma. The psychoeducational approach focuses on crisis intervention (Brock, Lazarus, & Jimerson, 2002; Brock, Sandoval, & Lewis, 2001; Poland, 1994) by preplanning and then implementing immediate interventions in the school setting in the first hours and days following a major crisis. The other, more clinical approach treats children who are identified as symptomatic at least one month after the traumatic event (Greenwald, 2000; Chemtob, Nakashima, & Carlson, 2002; Eth, 2001).

We believe that a comprehensive, continuous health-oriented approach should flexibly address various needs at different phases of coping with disaster and trauma. Thus, our book attempts to integrate the strengths of both preventative-immediate and long-term clinical interventions. We will delineate the spectrum of interventions that may fill the existing gap in intervention practice between immediate crisis interventions and later referrals for treatment when a full-blown symptomatic picture manifests itself months after the event. Our multisystemic, dynamic, psychoeducational approach underscores the best ways to strengthen the individual child's existing inner resources and to enlist the resources available in the child's multiple significant support systems.

Section B

The Psychological Impact of Disasters on Children

A ny disaster is a *potentially traumatic event*. The term *trauma* has both a medical and a psychological definition. Medically, trauma refers to serious or critical bodily injury, wound, or shock. Psychologically, it refers to a direct or indirect (e.g., witnessing) experience that is sudden, perceived to be dangerous, emotionally painful, distressing, or shocking. Trauma often involves physical manifestations and may result in *lasting* mental and physical effects. A parsimonious definition equates mental trauma with the persistence of disabling distress, dysfunction, or vulnerability after danger is over and adversity subsides (Shalev, 2002).

Clinicians identify characteristic reactions to traumatic events as they typically develop over time. The immediate reaction to disaster may be numbness due to shock. This is an involuntary but normal response. The common denominator of ensuing disaster responses comprises feelings of intense fear, helplessness, loss of control, and threat of annihilation. The event's impact generally induces distress regardless of individuals' premorbid or earlier experience, and it thus leads to stress responses regardless of one's prior level of functioning (American Academy of Pediatrics, Work Group on Disaster [AAPWGD], 1995; American Psychological Association [APA], 1980). These *normal responses* require substantial, often sustained, coping over some time; but the majority of people possess an adaptive coping capacity that enables them to overcome and accept their experience. However, if the traumatic experience is blocked out and not worked through, this may jeopardize the individual's (or organization's) ability to cope successfully. This, in turn, may lead to personal or organizational destabilization, which invokes a heightened sense of helplessness and lack of control. Consequences of this progression in individuals may lead to the disorders known as *acute stress disorder* (*ASD*) and *posttraumatic stress disorder* (*PTSD*). An event is deemed traumatic when it overwhelms

17

an individual's defenses and ability to react effectively, and when its effects do not disappear after a short time. The traumatic event then usually induces extreme anxiety or grief reactions. The individual feels emotionally, cognitively, and physically overwhelmed for a long duration.

A disaster may or may not cause adverse effects. Risk mechanisms involve a complex range of factors present before, during, and after the event. In this section of the book, we will first describe the magnitude and breadth of disasters' psychological effects, including contextual, personal, and recovery environment factors. Interventionists' awareness of the prevalence and combination of these factors will enable the identification of populations or groups with a relatively high likelihood of demonstrating postdisaster distress symptoms and disorders. At the end of this section, we will outline issues relevant to two of the most debilitating disasters of deliberate human origin.

Chapter 3

Impact of Context, Personal Factors, and Recovery Environment on Psychological Responses to Disaster

In recent years, much concern has developed among mental health professionals and educators regarding the effect of disasters on children, adolescents, schools, and communities in general (e.g., Brock, Lazarus, & Jimerson, 2002; La Greca, Silverman, Vernberg, & Roberts, 2002; Saylor, 1993). To understand the impact of diverse elements on disaster's effects, we will next relate to three general sets of factors that may lead to adverse psychological reactions: contextual (event) characteristics, personal vulnerabilities, and postdisaster recovery environment factors.

CONTEXTUAL/EVENT CHARACTERISTICS

The context of a community disaster necessarily reflects a *broader scope* in comparison to stressors that occur on an individual basis (Compas & Epping, 1993) and has a *random effect* on innocent victims in a community. A community disaster is usually defined as a sudden, overwhelming event that involves the destruction of property, includes injury or loss of life, affects an entire community, and is shared by many children and their families (American Academy of Pediatrics, Work Group on Disasters [AAPWGD], 1995). The event's impact is sufficiently broad in scope to induce distress in a very large group of people. From a school organizational frame of reference, the immediate demands produced by a disaster exceed the capacity of both the school organization and its related community services to respond effectively. Contextual features that seem related to the extent of adverse psychological effects include the disaster category, the event's intensity and scope, proximity to the event, the

duration and recurrence of traumatic exposure, situation-specific characteristics, mass media involvement, and loss of resources due to the traumatic event.

Disaster Category

Natural disasters may be differentiated from two types of human-related
disaster: accidental and deliberate human disasters. *Natural disasters*
encompass events such as earthquakes, wildfires, floods, and severe
storms. *Accidental human disasters* involve technology-based accidents or
catastrophes, such as mass transportation accidents, environmental con-
taminations (e.g., hazardous material spills), nuclear accidents, or dam col-
lapses. *Deliberate human disasters* entail acts of violence caused intentionally
by human beings, such as school shootings, hostage takings, terrorist acts,
violent civil disturbances, ethnic cleansing, and wars. This distinction
between the disaster categories is somewhat arbitrary. Occasionally, poor
preparation, the lack of preventive measures, faulty management policies,
corruption, and/or human errors contribute substantially to the impact of
technological and even natural disasters (e.g., homes built in unsafe flood-
prone areas, or faulty construction that increases the number of casualties
in an earthquake). Nevertheless, it appears that, generally, the two types
of person-related incidents arouse more psychological difficulty than do
natural disasters, which victims may perceive as "out of their hands" or
as "acts of God." Indeed, psychiatric disorders related to disasters are
likely to be more serious and persistent when resulting from an event
caused by other persons than from those resulting from non-human causes
(American Psychiatric Association, 2000). Moreover, the psychological
consequences of intentionally inflicted disasters are likely to be greater
than those of unintentional technological or natural disasters. The victims'
struggle to make sense of and find meaning for the disaster – a central
tool in processing and coping with it – may be compounded by the fact
that the disasters stemmed from deliberate and often indiscriminant
malicious, violent human acts.
    A special case of deliberate human disaster is politically inspired terror-
ism, whose very purpose consists of inflicting psychological pain. This
kind of terrorism aims to achieve a political goal by intentionally creating
collective fear, a sense of disequilibrium, and a perception of personal,
community, and governmental vulnerability. In such cases, more than in
natural or accidental disasters, the long-term personal safety issues and
the ability to trust others may comprise the salient treatment foci. Indeed,
war and terrorism, particularly when they become chronic conditions
without discrete beginning and end points, may be considered the worst
type of deliberate human disaster.

The Link between Disaster Category and Severity of Stress Responses

There is no evidence to suggest that the severity of children's responses varies across different types of natural disaster. However, certain symptoms may be more prevalent in response to specific disasters than to others. For example, survivors of hurricanes more frequently reported reexperiencing in the form of intrusive thoughts or dreams about the disaster than did survivors of other natural disasters (La Greca & Prinstein, 2002). With regard to accidental technological disasters, studies of large-scale transportation accidents with schoolchildren indicate a high incidence of both PTSD symptoms and other serious mental health problems in the first few weeks, including specific fears of traveling (Yule, Udwin, & Bolton, 2002). With regard to deliberate human disasters, studies have reported considerable effects of mass shooting episodes on victims; however, the prevalence rate of full-blown PTSD varies greatly. Survivors of certain disasters (e.g., flood-prone areas, radiation, toxic waste, terror attacks) may experience significantly longer periods of psychological distress, possibly due to the chronic stress associated with the unknown physiological consequences or continuing to live in or near a threatening environment. However, even in these cases, psychological symptoms decrease significantly over time (Salzer & Bickman, 1999). Victims of extreme terrorists' personal victimization may demonstrate severe and longer lasting symptomatology. Children directly involved may show trauma-related symptoms for years. The long-term effect of traumatic experience emerged, for example, in the case of a hostage taking of Israeli adolescents during a school outing. Survivors were studied 17 years after their face-to-face encounter with the terrorists, which included mass casualties. Most survivors reported some forms of traumata-related symptoms even 17 years after the terrorist assault (Desivilya, Gal, & Ayalon, 1996a, 1996b).

The Event's Intensity and Scope

The *intensity and scope* of a disastrous event comprise key factors in predicting schoolchildren's psychological reactions. A more terrifying or extreme event increases the likelihood that children will develop adverse psychological effects. Event-related contributors to severity of impact may include the degree of terror (e.g., threat of bodily harm) and horror (e.g., grotesque, morbid scenes), suddenness of onset, duration, degree of property damage, and the number of casualties.

Research has demonstrated that the experience of terror and personal danger correlates highly with the later emergence of PTSD symptomatology. Children's greater perceptions of threat to their lives and the lives of their loved ones correspond with higher reports of posttraumatic symptoms (Silverman & La Greca, 2002; McFarlane, 1992). Children experience the death or injury of a significant other – a parent, friend, teacher, classmate, or pet – as especially traumatic. In such cases, as described below in Chapter 6, posttrauma symptoms may mask, inhibit, and delay the grief work; thus, the traumatic part may require processing first, to allow the process of grief to continue its course (Raphael, Middleton, Martinic, & Misso, 1993). Factors that further complicate the grief and recovery processes include the children's struggle to reconcile why they survived but the loved ones did not, and children's ruminations regarding whether they could have done more to prevent the death from occurring in the first place (Silverman & La Greca, 2002). Children are at additional risk when their parents were similarly exposed and seriously affected, because effective parenting is potentially compromised (Almqvist & Brandell-Forsberg, 1995).

Proximity to the Event

Another factor placing children at greater risk for emotional injury following a traumatic event comprises the child's proximity to the incident (Pynoos & Nader, 1988). Proximity may include physical/geographical closeness to the critical incident, social proximity (membership in the same school body or afterschool club), and psychological proximity to the victim (a close relative or friend versus an acquaintance). Survivors with higher proximity to the disaster agent will likely demonstrate higher rates of post-event psychological disorders than will individuals with lower proximity. For example, a higher PTSD prevalence emerged among persons living in the area closest to the 2001 WTC attacks and among those who lost possessions than among other groups with less direct exposure (Galea et al., 2002).

In many cases, proximity appears to involve both physical and emotional aspects. For example, in a study of children exposed to missile attacks during the 1991 Persian Gulf War, predictors of stress included both distance from the areas hit by missiles and relative acquaintance with the injured victims (Schwarzwald, Weisenberg, Waysman, Solomon, & Klingman, 1993). Nevertheless, these two aspects of proximity may work separately at times; for example, in a study of seventh graders in a catastrophic bus accident, friendship with victims contributed uniquely to stress, as distinct from personal exposure (Milgram, Toubiana, Klingman, Raviv, & Goldstein, 1988).

In addition, children who have no direct contact with either the event or its victims may also be affected. This may occur via exposure to extensive media coverage or even merely hearing about a traumatic incident, which can lead to a strong feeling of identification with the affected community. For example, after a school shooting, students as well as staff members in neighboring schools may perceive themselves to be potential victims and may experience an acute trauma response. Twenty percent of a sample of children attending a middle school located 100 miles from the site of the 1995 Oklahoma City terrorist bombing, who had no direct physical or personal exposure to the incident, reported postdisaster symptoms that impaired their functioning at home or at school as much as two years later (Pfefferbaum et al., 2000).

A recently introduced term, *distant trauma*, relates to the response of those who did not personally undergo a threatening experience. Distant trauma comprises reactions (e.g., memory, thinking, symptoms) that are experienced at the time of a disastrous event, but from a remote and realistically safe distance (Terr et al., 1999). Terr et al.'s study on distant trauma in children after the Challenger spacecraft explosion in 1986 revealed that children's symptomatic patterns resembled PTSD and also several other symptoms not specified in the *Diagnostic and Statistical Manual of Mental Disorders* (*DSM III*; American Psychiatric Association, 1980). These additional symptoms consisted of trauma-specific fears (most common for both latency-aged children and adolescents), a fear of being left alone, and clinging to others (especially in children under age 10). In addition, adolescents evidenced diminished expectations for the future in general. Terr and her colleagues suggested that children who are raised from birth with television might perceive the immediacy of the medium almost as a reality.

In sum, proximity can be physical or geographical, but also psychological and social. As a consequence, the reactions of all those exposed, both directly and indirectly, must be observed for signs of emotional distress, as described below in Chapter 11 on preventive interventions.

Duration and Recurrence of Traumatic Exposure

Especially during a period of time in which no immediate relief is in sight, the *duration* of traumatic exposure may contribute to the intensity of stress reactions and be associated with a high risk for the development of PTSD. For children exposed to ongoing traumas, arousal symptoms may become modulated over time and reappear episodically (Realmuto, Masten, Carole & Hubbard, 1992).

Multiple exposures to traumatic events may also place children at higher risk. Symptoms found after single incidents may become more pronounced after multiple or prolonged events (e.g., war, prolonged captivity). Multiple exposures may place youngsters at higher risk for developing posttrauma symptoms, because children may merge similar incidents into a single representative memory (Howe, 1997). However, exposure to repeated traumatic incidents may plausibly lead to improved responding by providing some inoculation effects, by promoting stress reduction strategies, and by enhancing habituation. Thus, individuals who have competently resolved prior traumatic incidents may actually exhibit less distress and display greater competence when facing an additional traumatic event than will children exposed to only a single incident (Silverman & La Greca, 2002).

When living under *chronic conditions of continuous threat*, such as during wars, or the prolonged terrorism of the Palestinian uprising plaguing Israel since September 2000, changes in behavior, fears, and anxiety symptoms may be viewed as adaptive and even protective in reducing the risk of further exposure. A study conducted during a long period of recurrent terror attacks and shootings in Jerusalem (Pat-Horenczyk et al., 2003) revealed noted changes in the everyday routines of 12–16-year-old students who were not directly involved in any of the events. Of these adolescents, 57% reported a decrease in their number of outings downtown, about 33% reduced their number of visits to shopping malls, and 35% avoided nature hikes and/or travel by public transportation. Sixty-five percent reported fears focused on real dangers. These fears were not generalized to situations that did not represent a security risk at the time. Moreover, 95% of these adolescents reported no decline in academic or social functioning; most of the respondents continued their involvement in community and school life and rarely requested mental health assistance.

Although these situation-related behaviors call for mental health providers' special attention, in these unique circumstances the behaviors and symptoms per se do not necessarily comprise indications for referral to treatment. Unfortunately, at this point in time, neither qualitative nor quantitative longitudinal data exists to provide sufficient insight into the deeper levels of children's disaster-related psychological functioning and future mental health risk. The longer-term psychological cost of such exposure remains to be studied.

Situation-Specific Characteristics

Reactions to specific disasters may vary. For instance, after exposure to deliberate human violence, issues of human accountability, trustworthiness, and betrayal come to the fore, especially if a familiar individual perpetrated the act (Nader & Mello, 2002). Intentional violence perpetrated by terrorists shatters preschoolers' and elementary school children's trust in all adults. Particularly extreme reactions may arise, for example, from a school shooting carried out by a student from the same school. The similarity between aggressor and victim in these cases appears only to intensify feelings of betrayal and insecurity, such as in recent school shootings involving middle class assailants with neither criminal records nor other previously recognized risk factors found in high-density urban settings (Verlinden, Hersen, & Thomas, 2000).

Moreover, the very unexpectedness and randomness of such a situation in a familiar location (the school, local restaurant, or post office) may elicit prolonged concerns for personal safety. No one expects a young teenager (e.g., a 14-year old, as in the case of the 1999 Taber school shooting in Canada) to randomly gun down innocent students in a school's hallway, classroom, or cafeteria. Such an event strikes a blow to the morale and prestige of schools as a safe and caring place. Deliberate, random human brutality in an everyday setting may thus exacerbate the event's deleterious effect on developmental tasks such as developing morality or a sense of basic security and trust. It is thus essential that interventionists help children who experience such events to rebuild this broken trust, understand their psychological underpinnings and moral implications, and re-establish the security of familiar locations.

Other situation-specific reactions may typically include jitteriness, avoidance, guilt, anxiety, sleep disturbances, and so on. For example, following a loud terrorist shooting attack on an Israeli beachfront neighborhood, children evidenced perceptible reactions to noises; even the slight moving of a chair or the sound of a closing window increased tension dramatically (Klingman & Ben Eli, 1981). Nader and Mello (2002) described a similar example of a girl exposed to a school shooting who continued to freeze or jump for cover whenever she heard a loud bang, even after having moved to a safer community removed from the ongoing violence. Avoidance, guilt, and anxiety reactions may also emerge from specific situations. For instance, the aforementioned children exposed to the beachfront bombing completely avoided the site of the attack, despite its prior popularity as a social meeting spot (Klingman & Ben Eli, 1981). In another case, a teacher who ran for safety during a hostage taking later felt guilty for not running toward children to assist them; subsequently, the teacher could no longer jog daily for health and relaxation without thinking of the event (Nader & Mello, 2002). A specific event incurring anxiety reactions would be a delayed reunion with significant others (e.g., parents, siblings, close friends) during a community disaster. In such a case, children's natural anxiety about the welfare of these persons during the incident may later lead to isolated symptoms of separation anxiety that are specific to the persons of concern (Pynoos & Nader, 1988).

Mass Media Involvement

Disaster also inevitably attracts *mass media* attention. When the mass media highlight an event's random dramatic aspects – either destruction or heroism (i.e., a helpless victim or a "superhuman" rescuer) – viewers are usually denied a more balanced account of the event that would uncover the vast majority's active coping and resiliency. Victims find overblown media coverage to be irritating. Moreover, the constantly repeated images of dramatic scenes may have a hurtful impact on children and parents. Such coverage can result in distortions of facts (often unintentionally), an exaggerated focus on frightening dramatic sights, an overstating of the disaster's magnitude, and the perpetuation of disaster myths. As horrific as the news coverage might be, some children and their parents may be unable to resist viewing, thus, media exposure may reinforce feelings of vulnerability and fixate images of cruel death and destruction. Studies following the 1995 Oklahoma City terrorist bombing suggested that extensive television viewing may have contributed to an increase in PTSD symptoms (Pfefferbaum et al., 1999; Pfefferbaum et al., 2001).

Schools affected directly by dramatic violent events (e.g., a school shooting) attract a particularly inflated amount of mass media attention. Beyond the tendency for media coverage to sensationalize the event (Trump, 2000), there may be cases of naming, shaming, and blaming of schools by the media (especially in cases of fatal school violence), thereby placing the school's reputation at stake. After granting interviews with the media, children may later see or hear the interviews on television or radio (or hear about them from friends) and then feel overwhelmed with guilt for not providing the "desired" answers. Also, media focus on sensational details regarding the young perpetrators can contribute to copycat behaviors.

Loss of Resources

The final event-related contextual factor at play in responding to traumatic events comprises the loss of resources. By *resources* we refer to objects (e.g., home, school, clothing), conditions (e.g., position at work, social status), personal skills (e.g., social prowess, sense of personal efficacy), and energy resources (e.g., economic means).

Disaster may involve an immediate disruption in the functioning of infrastructures, as well as substantial long-term economic losses that affect families' resources and thus indirectly affect their children both during and long after the event. For example, recurrent terrorist attacks in Jerusalem caused a dramatic downfall in income from tourism, and local businesses collapsed due to shoppers' ensuing trepidation. Hurricanes constitute another example of disasters that cause widespread destruction; as a consequence, families may be uprooted from their neighborhoods, lose their homes and possessions, and must either rebuild or find new homes and possibly jobs elsewhere (Belter & Shannon, 1993; La Greca & Prinstein, 2002).

Loss of resources may constitute a critical ingredient in the stress response (Hobfoll, 2001). Research has shown that loss of possessions and damaged or destroyed infrastructures (e.g., community services) contribute to PTSD symptoms in children following disasters (Vernberg, La Greca, Silverman, & Prinstein, 1996). Displacement from home, school, and community may further intensify stress reactions. Forced dislocation and, especially, negative experiences in refugee camps (e.g., physical assaults, hunger, rape, and widespread infectious diseases) may produce additional adverse psychological effects. Resource loss can also be categorized into objective losses (e.g., of companionship, money, free time) and subjective losses (e.g., the feeling that things are not the same at school, the feeling that one is not important or valuable to others). One of the few studies on the influence of disaster-related resource loss on children (Asarnow et al., 1999) revealed that objective resource loss in the Northridge earthquake impacted children's postdisaster PTSD reactions.

PERSONAL CHARACTERISTICS

Aspects of children's functioning prior to disaster may influence their postdisaster reactions. Internal and relatively stable resilience and vulnerability factors play a role in both initial and long-term reactions to a psychological trauma. Individual characteristics comprise mental health history (e.g., preexisting psychopathology) and trauma history, personality factors, age, gender, and ethnicity and culture.

Mental Health and Trauma History

Some evidence indicates that a *preexisting mental disorder* (e.g., major depression and anxiety disorders) increases the risk of developing acute distress (Breslau, 1998) and may increase vulnerability to traumatic crisis (Nader & Pynoos, 1993). Preliminary findings suggest that, following a natural disaster, children with high levels of trait anxiety and those with a preexisting anxiety disorder are most likely to develop posttrauma symptomatology (e.g., Asarnow et al., 1999; Lonigan, Shannon, Taylor, Finch, & Sall, 1994). Trauma history, particularly an unsuccessfully resolved prior similar crisis, may also increase vulnerability to future traumatization.

Personality Factors

The fact that not all children develop chronic PTSD may indeed suggest the differentiating role played by personal vulnerability. However, the literature relating to children's trauma and personality is very limited. Trauma research presents methodological challenges regarding the unraveling of post-event reactions. It remains difficult to determine whether traits (e.g., insecurity) evidenced after a traumatic event represent preexisting factors that contributed to trauma vulnerability or represent a result of the trauma itself (Nader & Mello, 2002).

Personality factors may relate to many facets of responding to trauma. For example, emotional self-regulation, locus of control, faith or belief system, self-esteem, intellectual functioning, and temperament may all play a part. Contributing factors also include psychological resources such as coping style, including attitudes and beliefs that affect coping strategies, and self-efficacy or help seeking (Brock, 2002a, 2002b; Masten & Coatsworth, 1998).

In determining whether a particular event is or is not traumatic for a particular individual, one should consider the role of individuals' personal, subjective responses to life events as a determining factor. Constructivism (Kelly, 1955; Neimeyer, Keesee, & Fortner, 2000) views human beings as inveterate meaning makers who strive to punctuate, organize, and anticipate their engagement with the world by construing life events in terms of idiosyncratic systems of meaning organized around a set of core assumptions. Even intense initial responses such as fear, which is inherently biogenic, are also influenced by the survivor's subjective interpretation of the event, which, in turn, is influenced by previous experiences, coping skills, beliefs, and a variety of other factors. Ronen (1996) elaborated on the role of subjective reality in shaping children's responses to external events that adults considered traumatic. Constructivist therapy with traumatized children can target children's own major personal metaphors and narratives, allowing the child to find new meaning in the difficult experiences and learning to open up rather than to close down in the aftermath of trauma.

Chronological Age

In general, due to insufficient research, empiricists cannot yet generalize about children's vulnerability to stress reactions at different ages (Silverman & La Greca, 2002). However, with respect to symptomatology, developmentally-based variations appear in the extent and type of distress exhibited. Despite the substantial overlap of symptoms across age groups, general trends suggest the most frequently occurring reactions according to age group. As development is an individual process, the age group references below indicate only the typical symptoms that are more likely to appear within each age range.

Preschoolers and very young schoolchildren are generally more likely to exhibit marked postdisaster regressive behaviors such as unrelieved crying, excessive clinging and whining, thumb sucking, bedwetting, fears of darkness, separation, or being left alone, frightened facial expressions, somatic complaints, and immobility and/or aimless motion (National Institute of Mental Health [NIMH], 2000).

Elementary school children may have much the same regressive symptoms as preschoolers but also additional ones related to social interactions and to school studies. They may react to trauma with psychosomatic complaints, night terrors and other sleep disturbances, imaginary fears, withdrawal of interest in previously enjoyed peer activities, irritability, difficulty concentrating on schoolwork, a decline in academic performance, and outbursts of fighting, disobedience, and other aggressive behaviors (NIMH, 2000). Elementary school children may also develop distress, depression, or a preoccupation with the details of a traumatic event. Overall, preschoolers and younger elementary school children exhibit more specific fears and overt behaviors, whereas older elementary school children show more internalizing symptoms such as anxiety, distress, depression, and acute stress disorder.

As they approach junior high school, children become more competent in helping with their own recovery process, and their responses become increasingly adult-like. These responses include flashbacks, emotional numbing, nightmares, avoidance of any reminders of the event, depression, antisocial behavior, and difficulty with peers (NIMH, 2000). Preadolescents and adolescents may isolate themselves from family and friends, reveal emotional distress through somatic complaints, engage in more school truancy, and demonstrate mental confusion. They may move prematurely toward independence or increased dependence (Pynoos, 1990). Extreme guilt over failure to prevent injury or loss of life is often evidenced, resulting at times in vengeful thoughts that may interfere with the recovery process (Pfohl, Jimerson, & Lazarus, 2002). Adolescents may also show intense emotionality when the postdisaster circumstances cause cancellations or postponements of social events, or when teenagers' outings are restricted or strictly supervised by their parents. Often, childlike reactions appear alongside adult-like responses. Adolescents exhibit actual posttraumatic symptomatology that closely resembles that of adults.

These age-related differences may have their root in developmental differences in children's cognitive ability to comprehend the nature of traumatic events, and the age-related differences in coping repertoires. These differences have implications for intervention that are outlined in our discussion of special considerations (Chapter 10).

Gender Effects

Much research has shown that, irrespective of age, girls tend to report greater anxiety, more fears, more emotionality, and more PTSD symptoms than do boys. Two alternative explanations have emerged for these findings. One, it is possible that girls are more sensitive to threatening stimuli than boys, and, two, the more negative female reports may relate to masculine socialization patterns that prevent boys from reacting as openly as girls to potentially traumatic experiences and from reporting their negative emotions as freely (Klingman, Sagi, & Raviv, 1993). Some evidence suggests that boys tend to exhibit more externalizing symptoms and to report more behavioral and cognitive symptoms than do girls (Klingman et al., 1993; Pfohl et al., 2002). Another possibility to consider is that the type of trauma or disaster may affect gender differences; for example, boys may display more aggressive behaviors than girls when a disaster involves crime and intense violence (Gurwitch, Sitterle, Young, & Pfefferbaum, 2002). It should also be noted that when gender differences related to PTSD emerge, their magnitude is relatively modest and thus their clinical meaningfulness is uncertain (Vernberg et al., 1996).

In exploring adult gender-related behavior under conditions of stress, researchers recently suggested that although fight-or-flight may characterize the primary psychological response to stress for both males and females, females' responses show a more marked pattern of "tend-and-befriend" (Taylor et al., 2000). Tending involves nurturing activities designed to protect the self and offspring, which promote safety and reduce distress; befriending involves the creation and maintenance of social networks that may aid in this process. The behavioral mechanism that underlies the tend-and-befriend pattern under stressful circumstances appears to draw on the attachment caregiving system that depends, in part, on oxytocin, estrogen, and endogenous mechanisms, among other stress regulatory neuroendocrines (Taylor et al., 2000).

Ethnicity, Cultural, and Ideological Effects

Some research has suggested a relation between *membership in a minority group* and psychopathology (Fothergill, Maestas, & Darlington, 1999). Often, minority youth report higher levels of stress reactions and PTSD symptoms and exhibit more difficulties in recovering following a traumatic event. Hispanic ethnicity, for example, correlated with both PTSD and depression in a study conducted in Manhattan about two months after the 9/11 attacks (Galea et al., 2002). These associations may stem from a greater loss of resources, such as less financial backup or more inadequate insurance, or perhaps from different cultural patterns of expressiveness of negative emotions. Race and ethnicity may plausibly be markers for other variables, such as acculturation stress, prior traumas, stress from prejudices and discrimination, and cultural beliefs. However, it should be noted that other cultural factors, such as cultural ties and religious and other rituals, might protect against psychopathology (Rabalais, Ruggiero, & Scotti, 2002).

The perception of an event as traumatic depends not only on variables like psychological and material resources but also, for older children, on the individual's *beliefs and value systems*. Research suggests that ideology may contribute to adolescents' coping during war and politically violent situations (Klingman, 2002b; Punamaki, 1996). That is, political, national, or ideological affiliation may constitute an important factor in determining who is most affected. For instance, in the case of the assassination of the Israeli Prime Minister, Yitzhak Rabin, in 1995, young people experienced this politically violent event as more traumatic if they revealed closer psychological-ideological proximity to the victim (Raviv, Sadeh, Raviv, & Silverstein, 1998; Raviv, Sadeh, Raviv, Silverstein, & Diver, 2000). Evidence from the Israeli-Palestinian conflict, the Philippines, and South Africa suggests that ideological commitment to a political struggle and active engagement can be protective and increase adolescents' resilience. It is possible that the political meaning adolescents attribute to their traumatic experience leads them to interpret their symptoms as non-problematic (e.g., Kostelny & Garbarino, 1994; Punamaki, 1996). Thus, the way children (especially adolescents) make sense of a violent conflict (e.g., the causes of a war) may affect their mental health. However, when no opportunities exist for active engagement and the search for meaning only exposes adolescents to insoluble contradictions that lead to great psychological discomfort, affective disengagement may result in better psychological health (Jones, 2000).

THE POSTDISASTER RECOVERY ENVIRONMENT

Beyond contextual and personal variables, the role of the recovery environment constitutes the third major factor impacting children's functioning during and following disasters. Various facets of this environment's nature may encourage or impede the recovery process, including the extent to which that environment promotes a sense of safety, advances communality, encourages children's situation-specific adaptive coping, furnishes social support and fosters appropriate help seeking, entails adaptive psychological functioning of significant others, and attends to school organizational aspects.

Sense of Safety and Security

The child's immediate need following disaster is to feel safe; thus, a *sense of security and safety* in the immediate environment holds paramount importance for initial recovery. When emergency rescue workers evacuate children from a disaster site, the hospital emergency room staff, social workers, and others should make every effort to reunite these children with their families. A caring, reassuring attitude and gestures could have a marked impact on a frightened child at such times. Actions to ensure physically safe conditions and family reunification should be followed by psychoeducational efforts to reduce ongoing perceptions of threat, such as briefing children on the precautionary measures taken by governmental agencies, the family, the school, and establishments within the local community.

Sense of Communality

Next, children need a reconstructed *sense of community* that eventually decreases the negative impact of the adverse experience. *Communality* connotes an attachment to and concern about the community one lives in and is considered a contributing factor to various indicators of individual well-being (Davidson & Cotter, 1986). Researchers have attributed the finding of relatively low level stress responses after stressful situations in Israel to a sense of belonging in the community and to social cohesiveness (e.g., Klingman, 2000; Sagi, 1998; Ziv & Israeli, 1973). It is thus plausible that schoolchildren experience less stress in cohesive, nurturing classrooms in a caring school, where a shared sense of community exists, or is enhanced after a disaster through a variety of collective meaningful activities. These will be outlined in Part II of this book.

Situation-Specific Adaptive Coping

Children's coping efforts can be aided by their social milieu. Thus, a useful tool in the recovery process comprises systematic school-based efforts to *encourage situation-specific adaptive coping* skills in students. Toward this end, various authors have developed school-based intervention manuals that include activities designed to promote coping with community-wide traumatic events (e.g., American Red Cross, 2001; Gurwitch & Messenbaugh, 2001; La Greca, Vernberg, Silverman, Vogel, & Prinstein, 1994; Saltzman et al., 2002). These programs aim to serve as an immediate, school-based, on-site preventive intervention following disaster. Despite the limited well-designed research on these interventions' effectiveness, the programs derive from sound theoretical approaches and prior empirical findings on children, trauma, and disaster (Gurwitch et al., 2002). We will elaborate on such programs in Part II of the book.

Social Support and Help Seeking

Support persons and *support networks* provide a buffer against the psychological difficulties of traumatic experience. For children, three sources of support are available: familial, informal relationships like friendships, and formal relationships like those with teachers or mental health professionals. Younger schoolchildren, who depend on adults and on parental figures in particular, demonstrate great reliance on those figures for stress response cues, interpretations of traumatic events, a sense of security, and structural stability (see Chapter 7). Evidence for the importance of *family support* for children's coping with traumatic events can be gathered from studies examining adaptation following personal and community violence. Shepherd (1990) found that the amount of support that victims of personal violence received from their parents correlated inversely with the duration of victims' behavioral changes and mourning reactions. Similarly, Morrison (2000) reported that youngsters who lack family support demonstrate a higher risk for poor recovery following exposure to community violence.

Thus, the availability and perception of *social support* both play an important role in the recovery process. Perceived effectiveness of social support depends on one's evaluation of the accessibility and the prospective helpfulness of the support resource (Joseph, 1999; Kessler & McLeod, 1985). For example, for high school students exposed to violence, perceptions of an available supporter predicted fewer PTSD symptoms (Berman, Kurtines, Silverman, & Serafini, 1996). Research has shown that perceived social support from significant others mitigated the impact of natural disasters on children and adolescents (Venberg et al., 1996).

Children may not perceive all support persons as equally helpful, nor do they consistently explore all of the helper relationships available. *Help seeking* following disaster comprises a person-initiated response that may be either unmediated or mediated. Unmediated, automatic, unplanned help seeking is manifested in well-learned and well-established habits (e.g., turning to parents or teachers for soothing) that may or may not fit the current stressful circumstances. Mediated, cognitive help seeking involves a conscious appraisal of the current alternative social supports, to determine the best helper and the psychological cost-benefit ratio for seeking help in the given situation (Nadler, 1990).

In the wake of large-scale incidents, children found their parents to be more helpful than were teachers or any other support persons (e.g., Milgram & Toubiana, 1996: Klingman, 2001a). This preference for parental supports following large-scale traumatic events highlights the crucial importance of incorporating parents into comprehensive (multisystemic) school-based interventions. Age and personality factors may also influence help seeking behaviors. It is plausible that preschoolers and young elementary school children are more likely to use the automatic, unplanned route toward help seeking, especially when an unmediated external source of assistance (e.g., a significant other) is readily available. Older children, too, may engage in automatic help seeking, but, due to their growing attribution of importance to self-image and greater awareness of stigma, they may also initiate cognitive appraisal in their decision-making. Weisaeth (1995) has proposed that, in the wake of disaster, those with lower stress reaction levels are more likely to "go it alone" or to turn to familiar support figures for help; people with moderate levels consider turning to new as well as familiar support persons; and people with high stress levels consider turning to mental health professionals.

Once people regard certain support persons as helpful during the acute period of coping with a disaster and trauma, they will be more likely to search out or accept further help from these same people or people in these helpful categories. This "search and selection" process is presumed to characterize the behavior of children no less than that of adults (Milgram & Toubiana, 1996; Sarason, Sarason, & Pierce, 1995; Weisaeth, 1995). Thus, interventions should encourage both familial and within-school social supports, whether natural or formal.

Adaptive Psychological Functioning of Significant Others

In many cases of disaster, other members of the child's social milieu (e.g., parents, teachers, peers) may actually simultaneously undergo similar traumatic experiences and may experience either the same or a wider range of anxiety-related reactions. Considering the crucial impact on children of their *significant others' postdisaster psychological functioning and reactions*, we have devoted two separate chapters to this issue. For further discussion on the role of parents within the recovery environment, see Chapter 7, which expands on the effects of traumatic events on the family, the parent-child relationship, and the parent-school partnership. See Chapter 13 for a delineation of a range of interventions with parents.

School Organizational Aspects

The *organizational aspects* associated with the school may become crucial in helping with children's recovery. A mass disaster can disrupt the school's social structure and the associated social bonds. Chapter 11 elaborates on the many organizational steps to counteract the impact of trauma on the functioning of the school and its students.

Chapter 4

Two Extreme Contexts for Disaster: Terrorist Attack and Unconventional Weapon Use

Although the examples to follow represent cases of some of the most extreme deliberate human disastrous events, they also include features of other more common disasters and thus may enable readers insight into a variety of disasters. We next elaborate on two types of unpredictable events: one describing mass disasters that have already occurred around the world – terrorist attacks – and one examining the future threat of terrorism using unconventional means such as biological and chemical weapons.

TERRORIST ATTACKS

In general terms, terrorism involves the threat of politically inspired extraordinary violence with an intended impact broader than the immediate victim. The 1995 bombing of Oklahoma City's Alfred P. Murrah Federal Building represented the most deadly large-scale, single-incident, domestic terrorist act in the USA up to that date. Some of the ensuing research about how large-scale terrorism affects children who live in a country relatively free from large-scale, single-incident acts of violence (Gurwitch et al., 2002) demonstrated these acts' potentially serious psychological ramifications. Flynn (1996), Myers (2001), and Gidron (2002) reviewed those characteristics of terrorist-induced disasters that increase the magnitude and severity of psychological ill effects. These characteristics include terrorist acts' abrupt, sudden contrast to everyday reality, coupled with their particularly dramatic and gruesome disaster scenes that make the event all the more horrifying. Terrorism lacks warning, and disaster that strikes without warning produces maximum psychological and organizational disruption. The intentional human causality and the purposeful infliction of unspeakable pain and despair generate complicated and intense emotions such as anger, fear, and distrust of fellow human beings. In regions prone to repeated acts of terrorism over the long term, people develop an ongoing alert state infused with a sense of vulnerability, threat to personal safety, and intense, prolonged psychological symptoms. Throughout the community, widespread feelings of vulnerability, uncontrollability, and unpredictability emerge. Anxiety is intensified by individuals' and organizations' lack of familiarity with these types of events, how to prepare, and how to effectively respond. Civilians may feel that they have no way of preventing such future events, nor do the police, army, or government.

The *symbolism of targets* typifies terrorist acts. Such attacks seek out governmental agencies to weaken symbols of power. Attack of civilian public places conveys that no one is safe. This constellation of the deliberate human act, unexpectedness, heavy physical damage, and acute and chronic stressors elicits high levels of exasperation and rage across cultures. Organizations may be unprepared for their employees' intensity of emotions and reactions, which affect decision-making and operations.

UNCONVENTIONAL CHEMICAL, BIOLOGICAL, OR RADIOLOGICAL WEAPONS

Preparation for disaster at the beginning of this millennium must, unfortunately, take into account the threat of unconventional weapons in international as well as domestic terrorism. As the first millennium neared its end (i.e., the 1991 Gulf War), people around the world recognized the very real renewed threat posed by the use of chemical, biological, or radiological (CBR) weapons on civilian populations at the hands of extremists and terrorists. Fortunately, the Iraqi threat to devastate Israeli civilian areas, using long-range technologically advanced weapons capable of carrying chemical or biological warheads, was materialized neither during the 1991 Gulf War nor the recent 2003 war on Iraq. However, the danger of CBR stretches to other regions around the world. In 1995, a nerve agent was released on a Tokyo subway. That same year, USA authorities uncovered a terrorist effort to release a chlorine gas bomb in the Disneyland Theme Park in California, indicating that terrorist acts may be directly aimed at children. Repeated mailings of anthrax in the USA since 2001 have created heightened countrywide anxiety and alertness. Washington DC has been repeatedly warned of the probability of a "dirty bomb" attack (a conventional explosive used to disperse radioactive materials) in its metropolitan radius (Levine, 2003). In this section, we will discuss sources of fear concerning CBR; specific risks to children; secondary psychological effects of

CBR; practical and psychological difficulties in preparing for bio-chemical threat; and recommendations for preventative interventions.

Sources of Fear Concerning CBR

Considering the general population's unfamiliarity with CBR weapons and their effects, such a terrorist attack would likely produce a climate of grave uncertainty and insecurity that may intensify psychological risk. The threat of infection by an invisible, silent, odorless, humanly undetectable agent touches a deep human concern about the risk of being annihilated by a powerful, evil, imperceptible force, thus arousing emotions that cannot be straightforwardly eased by tools of reason (Holloway, Norwood, Fullerton, Engel, & Ursano, 1997; Stockes & Banderet, 1997). For most children, the microbial world is a terrifying mystery. Additionally, exposure to CBR carries *unknown, frightening health effects* on people's own present and future health and renders possible hidden damage to future generations. Continuous fears for one's safety and security can lead to feelings of vulnerability and powerlessness, overwhelm one's coping resources, and produce avoidance of thoughts and feelings associated with CBR. Long-term avoidance may, in turn, reduce opportunities to minimize or diminish fear responses through exposure to information about one's safety and invulnerability that could correct exaggerated beliefs (Yehuda, 2002).

Fear of the unknown can disrupt communities, as people tend to flee from a perceived danger zone or distance themselves physically and emotionally from those who have been exposed. When a sizable population shares a CBR threat, the belief that treatment will be provided to some but not to others may contribute to demoralization and possibly to societal disruption as people lose faith in major community institutions. In contrast to such scenarios, however, past observation of conventional disasters and disease outbreaks indicates a pattern of minimal civilian panic and, in the long run, generally effective and situation-adaptive collective responses (Glass & Schoch-Spana, 2002; Omer & Alon, 1994). Nevertheless, it is not known how the population would react to an unprecedented act of CBR terrorism; it is plausible that people would be reluctant to remain in a contaminated area, and panic reactions should be considered a possibility.

Specific Risks to Children

Presumably, as with other health risks, children would suffer more extreme effects from a chemical or biological weapon's release than would adults. For example, children's higher number of respirations per minute may result in exposure to a relatively greater dosage of aerosolized agents such as sarin, cyanide, or anthrax. Also, the high vapor density of some gases (e.g., sarin, chlorine) places their highest concentration close to the ground – in the lower breathing zone of children. The more permeable skin of children in conjunction with a larger surface-to-mass ratio would also result in greater exposure to transdermally absorbed toxicants. Moreover, because of their relatively larger body surface area, children lose heat quickly when showered, and shower decontamination in a cold climate may result in hypothermia. In addition, lower fluid reserves increase the child's risk of rapid dehydration or shock after vomiting and diarrhea. Vesicants and corrosives (e.g., mustard gas) also would produce greater injury to children because of their poor keratinization.

Beyond these direct health effects, children would also undergo augmented motor, cognitive, and psychological risks. Immature motor skills would reduce younger children's likelihood of escaping from a hazardous area. Younger children may not have the cognitive ability to comprehend danger or to decide when, where, and in which direction to flee. In mass casualty incidents, children who witness the weapons' effect (possibly on their parents) are also at risk for developing psychological injuries as a result of the experience (see also the Policy Statement that appeared in *Pediatrics*, 2000, pp. 662–670).

Secondary Psychological Effects of CBR

The invisibility of biological and chemical agents may lead to false-alarm reactions. After a Scud air missile attack on Israel during the 1991 Gulf War, feared exposure to chemical weapons caused nearly 700 of the 1000 war-related visits to emergency rooms (Bleich, Dycian, Koslowsky, Solomon, & Wiener, 1992). False alarms may be generated by the spread of rumors, the innocuous use of chemical and electronic detectors, authorities' use of protective suits for detection of unconventional agents, or people mistaking common bodily symptoms (e.g., due to minor infectious diseases, allergic reactions, stress and anxiety) and nonspecific symptoms (e.g., eye irritation, skin rashes) for early symptoms of CBR exposure. Psychogenic symptoms (e.g., hyperventilation, nausea, muscle tension, tremors, sweating) may be indistinguishable from early stages of CBR attack (Bartholomew & Wessely, 2002).

False alarms may result in a mass sociogenic episode affecting schools. In sociogenic episodes, members of a cohesive group experience a rapid spread of symptoms originating from a nervous system disturbance involving excitation and loss or alteration of functions, causing physical complaints that have no corresponding organic etiology. It seems that no particular predisposition exists for this behavioral reaction, which anyone can exhibit under certain circumstances. Symptoms are spread via sight, sound, or rumor; this spread occurs down the age scale, beginning in older or higher-status students, with a preponderance of female participants (Bartholomew & Wessely, 2002). Bartholomew and Wessely reviewed a number of such mass sociogenic cases involving schools and children. During political unrest in Soviet Georgia in 1989, symptoms spread among 400 adolescent females at several nearby schools after rumors spread that students were exposed to poison gas following the use of a conventional chemical agent chloropicrin to disperse a rally. In September 2001, paint fumes set off a bioterrorism scare at a middle school in Washington State, resulting in referrals of 16 students and a teacher to the hospital. In the following month, over 1000 students in several schools in Manila, Philippines deluged local clinics with mundane flue-like symptoms such as coughs, colds, and mild fever after rumors spread via short-text services that such symptoms were due to bioterrorism. That same year, a teacher and student reported minor forearm "chemical burns" after opening a letter and discerning a powder in the air; subsequent analysis revealed no foreign substance in the envelope (Lehman, 2001).

The social and psychological impact of mass sociogenic illness and associated anxiety may be as severe as that from a confirmed attack. Bartholomew and Wessely (2002) suggested that it might be advisable to close the school until negative test results confirm the area's safety. Importantly, closure temporarily disperses the group and thus limits the potential spread of symptoms. It also allows time for experts to determine whether the cases correspond with somatoform disorder and to assist in reducing anxiety levels.

In some cases of actual CBR, the effects can be more psychological than real. One such example is the case of the "dirty bomb." This type of bomb's conventional explosive would dilute its radioactivity, making it almost impossible for a person to receive a radiation dose sufficient to cause acute illness. Yet, such an attack would possibly cause noted civil disruption, necessitating evacuations to clean up contaminated areas, which could result in disproportional psychological responses. Swift information dissemination and education by crisis managers could substantially contain the collective panic, limiting its extent and duration and thus counteracting psychological damage. Children in particular must be educated about the difference between a nuclear bomb (which splits atoms to release tremendous amounts of energy and create radioactive materials) and the "dirty bomb."

Practical and Psychological Difficulties in Preparing for Bio-Chemical Threat

Anticipatory CBR activities may themselves be potentially traumatic. For example, in both the 1991 and 2003 Gulf Wars, soldier-teachers implemented a gas mask training program to school students throughout Israel in their classrooms. In weighing the benefits of preparation for unconventional warfare against the psychological cost of this intervention, the relevant governmental agencies realized this training would raise students' fears about an immediate outbreak of air strikes on Israel (founded in 1991, but not in 2003).

The logistical and emotional experiences that Israeli civilians underwent during the unprecedented 1991 war may help future intervention planners. Although all of the air missiles that fell in Israel during those weeks had conventional warheads, during the war itself the threat of biological or chemical attack was very real and imminent, as explained by governmental authorities and as seen in media broadcasts of Iraqi threats. Air missile attacks occurred sporadically during the night, sometimes more than once per night, and the mass media advised families each time to take cover in sealed rooms, don gas masks, and await announcements identifying the locations hit and the type of missile. Schools were closed down. Children and parents became hypervigilant concerning the warning sound of the wailing air-raid siren. After rushing into the sealed rooms, putting the protective gear on their children posed a challenge for many parents. Gas masks are uncomfortable, tend to fog, dry out the mouth, and have a frightening, alien or "inhuman" appearance for younger children. The rubber masks have an unpleasant smell, weight, and pressure and may cause difficulties breathing and communicating. Besides donning their own masks, parents needed to help younger children into hooded protective gear with air pumps; place toddlers and infants into protective infant carriers; and help older children adjust S-shaped metal clasps on four side straps.

In some cases, parents had to deal with a perceived real-life emergency of a child's refusal to use the gas mask. As a case illustration, one preschooler demonstrated temper tantrums, anger, and aggression when asked to don the mask. His parents' difficulty was complicated by their feelings of urgency and very high anxiety with regard to their geographical proximity to the hardest-hit area of central Israel. In this case, a family-based cognitive-behavioral intervention (Klingman, 1992) led to noted improvement within 3 days.

During those minutes, sometimes hours, inside the sealed rooms, parents waited anxiously for the all-clear signal. Those who heard sounds of missiles falling in their area waited to ascertain whether the missiles were unconventional. Parents had to attend to the children's anxiety as well as more prosaic concerns such as the children's boredom, all adding to their own anxiety and the exhaustion of around-the-clock care due to school closure. Children using protective measures often perspired greatly and became irritable in the small sealed rooms. Some people wore protective clothing, which is bulky and cumbersome and impedes physical agility in caring for small children and performing procedures such as venipuncture, if necessary.

Recommendations for Preventative Interventions

Considering the research on factors known to provoke and amplify worry, fear, helplessness, and anger in threatening situations, we can strongly argue that demystifying the world of CBR weapons will provide intervention planners with a key prevention measure. Age-related information dissemination and education comprise the crucial preventive measures to be handled by the schools, augmented by parent education. Schoolchildren should receive clear, practical instruction in how to follow personal protective measures and practices as well as information on the community and school's protective actions. Instruction in particular coping strategies (e.g., to be used while waiting in a sealed room to reinforce a sense of control) can help minimize panic and other adverse psychological effects (Klingman, 1992; Klingman & Kupermintz, 1994).

Concrete educational materials can offset preschoolers' fears and uncertainty raised by parents' and teachers' direct frontal explanations about the world of CBR. For example, in collaboration with expert kindergarten teachers and artists, Israeli school psychologists developed story-and-coloring booklets peopled by alien-like, amusing clown figures visiting a cave in space where the air is polluted, and also a teddy bear for which the young child prepares a gas mask and must deal with the teddy's anxiety (Klingman, 2002c).

SUMMARY

We have demonstrated through our examination of the unique characteristics of two types of disasters – terrorist attacks and the future threat of terrorism using unconventional weapons – how each disaster presents unique risks and challenges, both in the physical as well as in the psychological realms. We have shown how familiarity with such characteristics offers many implications for prevention. These specific disasters may also help clarify general processes of reacting to, coping with, and processing of trauma for different types of disaster and traumatic loss, as will be outlined in the next section.

Postdisaster Stress and Loss Reactions, Processing, and Coping

T his section examines how children, and the adults around them, react to a disaster. The first chapter in this section describes the continuum of postdisaster stress reactions, ranging from normative transient responses and symptoms up to full-fledged, long-lasting PTSD. We then elaborate on the specific case of traumatic loss and bereavement. Next, the familial complex chain of reactions is explored. Last, special consideration is given to coping, positive adaptational, and growth reactions.

Chapter 5

From Normative Postdisaster Stress Response to Full-Fledged Disorder

Postdisaster stress reactions can be divided into two broad categories. One relates to postdisaster stress *responses* during the first month, which range from normal, very short-lived stress reactions to a transient acute stress disorder (ASD) that often passes without leaving pathological residuals. The other relates to long-lasting diagnosable pathological *disorders*, in particular to posttraumatic stress disorder (PTSD), depression, and anxiety disorder.

NORMATIVE POSTDISASTER STRESS RESPONSE

Any unexpected novelty incongruent with previous life experience triggers a process of adjustment and adaptation. The novelties experienced during disasters may be among the most unspeakable, horrific experiences known to humankind. Children may experience an immediate threat to their own lives (e.g., being trapped or held hostage) or personal injury; they may witness the inescapable horror of others' mutilation, torture, or death; and they may face deliberate human malevolence, the loss of loved ones, the loss of possessions, forced dislocation, and uncertainty about the future. Strong physiological, cognitive, and emotional responses comprise normal reactions to such extremely adverse situations. Survivors nearly universally express early psychological and biological symptoms that in most cases are socially acceptable. Such reactions imply a natural, normal, functional, and adaptive process of working through the experience. The process of working through the traumatic experience does not imply that children do not suffer temporarily from symptoms; most children will struggle with some psychological and/or physical ailments but will recover without professional help. Such symptoms should not, however, be regarded as comprising a "disorder" unless they significantly interfere with recovery and functioning.

Following exposure to a disaster, many children find they are acting in unexpected and unfamiliar ways, some of which may indeed resemble symptoms of a disorder. Victims' emotional reactions vary. Heightened arousal is manifested as feelings of anxiety accompanied by physiological arousal and by engagement in excessive activity. Feelings of fear, helplessness, and powerlessness dominate. Psychic numbing may appear as feelings of being stunned, dazed, confused, disorganized, and apathetic or sensing an automaton-like carrying out of daily activities, along with the denial of events and their impact. These behaviors, which are mostly transient, may reflect cognitive distortions in response to trauma and, for some, may indicate a level of dissociation.

Relatively little empirical data exists pertaining to children and adolescents' reactions immediately after a traumatic event. Reports have described psychological reactions that can in general be described as *psychic shock*: disbelief, a sense of strangeness, feeling stunned and overwhelmed. Youngsters view community disaster as outside the realm of normal human experience; expressing colloquial reactions to disaster like: "It was surreal" or "It felt like I was in a movie."

After the initial shock, children will likely feel the need to vent their emotions, so as to take stock and begin to cope with the anxieties they could not handle at the time of impact. Other types of common emotional responses include diffused anxiety (e.g., exaggerated startle response, inability to relax, clinging to loved ones), survivor guilt (e.g., feeling responsible for the unfortunate fate of others), and grief reactions to loss. Some may strongly feel the need to be with others at all times. Some may be dependent on others yet suspicious, and may feel no one can understand what they have been through. Others may feel a need to distance themselves emotionally from others and may be irritable in the face of sympathy. Some may shift from one kind of response to another. Sadness, anger, and hopelessness may be evident, as well as contrary feelings of elation as a result of survival relief or involvement in the rescue efforts. Insomnia or nightmares may appear. The physiological reactions can be described in terms of Selye's (1956) "general adaptation syndrome," but this aspect of children's reactions has not been well studied (Silverman & La Greca, 2002).

In general, clinicians consider all these trauma-related reactions to be normal. Most children, in the days and weeks following the disaster, show a progressive decline in symptoms rather than developing PTSD; they typically cope with the new situation and recover quickly. The immediate post-event stress response can thus be conceptualized as a short-term, transient, normal reaction to abnormal circumstances – symptoms that do not necessarily predict a disorder. Early symptoms may even play an adaptive role. Such symptoms may effectively communicate the child's need for help, recruit support, and also enhance a sense of togetherness. Moreover, acknowledging these early symptoms may assist the child in attending to the situation and its consequences, thereby enabling deeper mental processing of the traumatic experiences. Such normative processing of events – *working through* – may include verbalizing bodily and sensory experiences, recalling memories, reappraising events, and forming coherent understandable narratives of the events. Indeed, the ability to successfully process the adverse experience independently, without professional help, may empower survivors. Hence, interventionists should keep in mind that some forms of individualized treatments may possibly be delivered too early and interfere with normal processing.

Nevertheless, for some children and adolescents, the struggle to process a disaster lasts much longer, is blocked, or escalates until symptoms become a source of significant distress and a decline occurs in social, familial, academic, or occupational performance. Only when children's symptoms become highly intense, pervasive, and generalized or prolonged (e.g., nightmares continue, recollections remain fragmented and poorly verbalized, fears become generalized) may they signal a risk for the development of a disorder, indicating the need for more specific individualized interventions. The distress may manifest itself in more intense and prolonged psychological and physiological reactivity that interferes with the child's ability to cope with post-event reactions and may also underlie avoidance behavior. For example, children may restrict certain activities to avoid confronting reminders that strongly evoke trauma-related images. In such cases, if symptoms are not addressed and resolved relatively quickly, they may interfere with the natural recovery process and may then develop into a disorder (Brom & Kleber, 1989). The appearance of any of three specific phenomena immediately after the event – dissociation, depression, or a full-blown syndrome of ASD (see below) – indicate possible future difficulties and require a rather early clinical intervention.

Explanatory Models for the Development of Normative Early Stress Reactions

Various theoretical models may explain normative stress responses to disaster. Learning theory explicates the excessive arousal and acute distress associated with trauma in terms of classical conditioning. Fear and anxiety relevant to the context of the trauma are generalized to similar situations. This may lead to avoidance of feared situations and to reinforcement of the conditioned response. Another explanation, suggested by the limbic appraisal hypothesis within the neuropsychological model of information processing (Hartman & Burgess, 1993), asserts that stimuli are first processed by the limbic system before being transmitted to the neocortex where reactions are interpreted. If the limbic system is overwhelmed, the routing of information may be comprised by deregulation in the limbic system, which affects the meaning systems. When not resolved, the event remains in active memory or becomes defended by cognitive mechanisms (like denial) that result in fragmented memory and reexperiencing of the trauma.

Another explanatory model asserts that a disastrous event places demands on the individual to process information that challenges core beliefs such as that the world is benign and meaningful, that people are trustworthy, and that the self is worthy (Janoff-Bulman, 1992). In general, people perceive themselves as indestructible and invulnerable to victimization. The traumatic experience *shatters fundamental assumptions* that normally go unquestioned and unchallenged – about the positive value and agency of the self, trust in others, the safety of the world, and the meaning of life. Having an inherent need to integrate the many facets of the traumatic event into a more coherent whole within their self-structure, survivors begin the search for meaning and for a sense of control and predictability. Emotional processing, that is, reconciling the traumatic experience with these beliefs, is necessary for recovery. In this sense, coping involves reexamining issues of safety, caring, responsibility, and trust; adjusting at least some old assumptions; and accepting some new (or less positive or idealistic) beliefs, thus "rebuilding" the inner world and reestablishing meaning. Presumably, effective coping from this perspective would integrate the adverse event into broader, positively meaningful structures rather than focusing on the malevolence of the world around. Often, these coping efforts include spiritual or religious avenues to meaning-making (see Chapter 12). Eventually, over time, most survivors reestablish an assumptive world that is less threatening. The process is a dynamic one, of working through the experience of disruption and powerlessness. Continued psychological difficulties in processing may indicate ineffective processing of the information that challenges core beliefs. Rather, the traumatic experience is represented in memory in such way that it increases stress (e.g., the world is dangerous; I cannot control what happens to me), and this further interferes with the processing of the traumatic event.

POSTTRAUMATIC STRESS DISORDER (PTSD) IN ADULTS AND CHILDREN

Along the continuum from normative transient stress reactions to long-lasting diagnosable mental disorders following a disaster, PTSD comprises the fullest, most commonly researched trauma-related disorder. This disorder consists of a specific manifestation of trauma-related destabilization. PTSD can only be diagnosed if the individual demonstrates a specific cluster of symptoms at least one month after exposure to a traumatic event. The disorder can manifest itself differently in children and adults.

Diagnostic Criteria for PTSD

To satisfy criteria for PTSD (American Psychiatric Association, 1994, 2000), individuals must have been exposed to a traumatic event (criterion A) in which they experienced, witnessed, or learned about a significant other's exposure to an unexpected event or events that involved actual or threatened death or serious injury, or a threat to the physical integrity of the self or others. The individual must also have responded with intense fear, helplessness, or horror to meet criteria for a PTSD diagnosis. Children, however, may express agitated or disorganized behavior rather than fear or helplessness.

Three clusters of symptoms (criteria B, C, and D) must be present. These symptoms must persist for at least one month after the trauma (criterion E) and significantly interfere with the individual's functioning (criterion F). Symptoms may appear immediately after, or days after, or several weeks after the traumatic event; in a small proportion of the population symptoms may emerge more than six months after the event (i.e., delayed onset).

For diagnosis, the person must exhibit at least one of the reexperiencing symptoms comprising the *first symptom cluster* (criterion B). These include intrusive memories (e.g., unwanted distressing recollections of the incident), flashbacks, distressing dreams of the event, a sense of reliving the trauma, and psychological distress or physiological reactivity when reminded of the trauma by internal or external cues. Younger children may experience distressing dreams of the event that may change within several weeks into generalized nightmares of monsters, of rescuing others, or of threats to self or others, and there may be frightening dreams without recognizable content. Intrusive memories may also find expression in children's repetitive play, reliving of the event, or reenactments in play that express themes or aspects of the event.

The *second cluster* of symptoms (criterion C) refers to attempts to avoid reminders of the critical event, including stimuli associated with the event and numbing of general responsiveness. For diagnosis, the person must exhibit at least three of the following: persistent avoidance of thoughts, feelings, and reminders of the trauma; inability to recall some aspects of the trauma; estrangement from others and diminished interest in normal activities, emotional numbing; and a sense of foreshortened future.

The third cluster (criterion D) refers to persistent symptoms of heightened arousal that reflects a state of constant preparedness for danger. For diagnosis, the person must experience at least two of the following: insomnia, irritability, impaired concentration, anger, hypervigilance, or an exaggerated startle response.

Although some studies of children and adolescents have, to a large extent, replicated the PTSD findings of adult populations (Bolton, O'Ryan, Udwin, Boyle, & Yule, 2000), others have purported the inadequacy of these criteria for children (See Chapter 14 for a detailed discussion.) Children are more likely to manifest their distress as behavioral problems, school difficulties, school absenteeism, new separation anxiety, aggression, and regressive behaviors.

Prevalence and Course of PTSD

Very few epidemiological and longitudinal studies have thoroughly investigated the prevalence of PTSD among children and adolescents following a community or a school disaster. Among these, the findings are inconsistent, showing rates within one year of the trauma ranging from 5% to 90% (American Academy of Child and Adolescent Psychiatry [AACAP], 1998; Korol, Kramer, Grace, & Green, 2002; Trappler & Friedman, 1996). Nevertheless, most experts agree that larger numbers of children and adolescents than previously suspected experience significant disaster-related symptomatology and behavior changes for months after a disaster's initial impact and that up to a third of the young people in a community may develop PTSD following a community disaster (Yule, Perrin, & Smith, 2000). Findings of several studies suggest that once a child develops full-blown PTSD, the difficulties are likely to be severe, to follow a chronic course, and to be difficult to resolve even with treatment (Gurwitch, Sitterle, Young, & Pfefferbaum, 2002). However, literature reviews of the long-term effects of community trauma (with special reference to children and adolescents) reveal that only a small number of affected children experience the trauma as a significant turning point after which effects are difficult to reverse (e.g., Saigh, Green, & Korol, 1996; Salzer & Bickman, 1999).

Explanatory Models for the Development of PTSD

PTSD appears to represent a failure to recover naturally from a nearly universal set of emotions and reactions. Symptoms such as hypervigilance, dissociation, avoidance, and numbing exemplify coping strategies that may have been functional and effective at the time of the event but later interfere with the individual's adaptation. Studies of the *biological mechanisms* of PTSD have delineated circumscribed alternations in brain regions, such as the amygdala and hippocampus, which correspond with fear and traumatic memory as well as with changes in hormonal, neurochemical, and physiological systems involved in coordinating the body's response to stress. Psychological and biological data support the hypothesis that a failure to contain the biological stress response at the time of the trauma facilitates the development of PTSD. This failure results in a cascade of alternations that lead to intrusive recollections of the event, avoidance of reminders of the event, and symptoms of hyperarousal

(Yehuda, 2002). Hence, victims suffer from fragmented, somatic, and affective recalling of their trauma (van der Kolk & Fisler, 1995).

Foa and her colleagues (e. g., Foa & Meadows, 1997) provided an *information processing theory* for PTSD to explain such symptoms as intrusive thoughts and avoidance. They postulated that information related to the traumatic events is stored in "fear networks" in the brain; circuits in the fear network are activated by trauma-related stimuli, and these circuits try to suppress the information when it threatens to enter into consciousness. To resolve the trauma, information in the fear network must be assimilated into existing memory structures.

ACUTE STRESS DISORDER

The *DSM-IV* (American Psychiatric Association, 1994) later added another disaster-related diagnosis that closely resembles PTSD but has an earlier onset and shorter duration. Acute stress disorder (ASD) refers to trauma reactions that occur within the first month following the traumatic event, lasting for a minimum of two days and a maximum of four weeks Although PTSD and ASD share an overlap of many symptoms, ASD differs in its main emphasis on dissociative symptoms. For diagnosis, the person must evidence at least three of the following five symptoms: emotional numbing, reduced awareness of one's surroundings, derealization, depersonalization, or dissociative amnesia.

Although PTSD does not always ensue following ASD, the latter diagnosis can pinpoint individuals who evidence high risk for subsequent development of PTSD. However, the appearance of acute stress symptoms within the first few days or weeks following a disaster does not necessarily predict long-term maladjustment. Before ASD can be applied to children as a predictor of PTSD, prospective studies must be conducted with children at different developmental stages (Salmon & Bryant, 2002). Because the prospective course of PTSD in children may differ from that of adults, particularly with respect to the emphasis on dissociation, the assessment and treatment of ASD in children remains very much similar to that of PTSD (DeBellis, 1997).

SUBCLINICAL OR OTHER PATHOLOGICAL DISORDERS

Many children directly exposed to trauma do not meet the full criteria for either ASD or PTSD. Nevertheless, many report some symptoms like reexperiencing of the trauma, avoidance of situations related to the trauma, or a state of hypervigilance (e.g., Klingman, 2001a). A vivid illustration of such partial PTSD symptomatology emerges from a newspaper interview with a 19-year-old Israeli who was wounded in a terrorist attack on a shopping mall 5 years earlier (Rotem, 2002). She reported that her life had "changed tracks" after the attack: She shows many avoidance and fear reactions like avoiding buses and restaurants and keeping away from crowded places, and when outside her home, she constantly checks who is in front of her and who is behind her, to espy possible terrorists. However, she claims, "It is not so dramatic as it sounds. I live with it, I have adjusted well to this, and I cannot remember how it was to live without constant fear; I live like anyone who has learned to walk on crutches."

Research also indicates that other psychiatric disorders such as major depression and anxiety disorders may accompany PTSD in disaster survivors, especially following disasters that involved the loss of loved ones (for an extended review, see Silverman & La Greca, 2002; Vernberg & Varela, 2001).

Chapter 6

Bereavement in the Wake of Traumatic Death

Community disasters involve forcible losses of loved ones, close members of the family, schoolmates and friends, or teachers, not to mention the losses of pets and destroyed homes or classrooms. The grief process that follows comprises, in most cases, part of the healing process. However, in some cases, especially for adolescents, the grief process can be an isolating experience dealt with slowly or in intermittent outbursts. In any case, during this process the child cannot remain passive and simply wait for things to get better. The child must complete certain tasks such as understanding the permanence of death, expressing and processing feelings, attaining emotional acceptance, commemorating, assimilating the loss, and moving on. The particularly traumatic circumstances surrounding the losses incurred during disaster are likely to compound the recovery process. This chapter will discuss the bereavement process, developmental aspects in the grief process, and the particular difficulties inherent in losses caused by disastrous events.

THE BEREAVEMENT PROCESS

Parkes (1996) reported that, during the first year of bereavement, grieving adults often attempt to deny the reality of the loss and search for the lost person, attempt a reunion in dreams and fantasies, and experience anger, pangs of emotional pain, tearfulness, sadness, and depression. Based on a one-year follow-up study following a school ground sniper attack, elementary school students demonstrated a grief response similar to that of adults, both in the nature and the frequency of grief reactions (Pynoos & Nader, 1988). Although grief expression is unique to each individual, certain commonalties exist, in line with the bereavement phases devised by

Bowlby (1961), Parkes (1996), and Horowitz (1976). Although initially presented as phases, they do not always follow in sequence, and they commonly repeat and overlap; thus, a better term may be *process components.* These components consist of:

1. *Shock and denial.* The instinctive responses when first confronting the death of a loved one may involve feelings of numbness, difficulty in fully realizing what has happened, internal attempts to act as if the event did not occur, or attempts to make believe that the deceased will return.

2. *Protest, yearning, bargaining, and intrusion.* The second component in the grief process involves preoccupation with the deceased and with places and things that arouse memories of the deceased. This component may include angry protest toward the deceased or other people, often seemingly without cause. It also includes yearning, longing, and searching for the deceased and may involve bargaining, mostly with God (e.g., the child may offer to "do things for God" if God will bring the loved one back). Often a child will feel some responsibility for the death (e.g., because of prior arguments, anger, or a "death wish") or guilt feelings because of prior behavior or "unfinished business" with the deceased. Unwanted intrusive reexperiencing of parts of the event may occur, combined with hypervigilance. All these may result in temporarily turning inward.

3. *From disorganization and despair to working through.* The mourner gradually recognizes the reality of the loss. This involves acceptance, detachment, and reorganization. The relative investment in daily life increases, openness to outside stimulation is regained, a certain degree of disengagement from the deceased occurs, and eventually new relations can be established.

These three process components comprise a normal process of adapting emotionally, cognitively, and behaviorally to the loss. The length of the adjustment period and the specific nature of responses vary. They depend on individual characteristics of the bereaved (including coping style and coping skills), the nature of the relationship with the deceased, demographic factors (e. g., age, gender, socioeconomic status), the circumstances of death, cultural factors, and the quality and availability of natural support systems. For some people, the grief process may take months, for others even years. A "normal" mourning period may last one to two years, but feelings of sorrow at the loss last much longer, perhaps forever.

Clinicians consider grief or bereavement as a cause for concern only when the intensity of grief is so overwhelming that symptoms are acute and unmanageably intense, or when one has difficulty moving along this working-through process. The exaggerated and distorted expression of grief (both in duration and intensity) that affects the person's functioning and delays adaptation may be termed: "unfinished grief," "unresolved grief," "reactive depression," "pathological mourning," and, more recently, "complicated grief." *Complicated grief* may be explained as "frozen blocks of time," whereby life issues remain unexpressed or unacknowledged and the normal grief process stops, thus denying the person a natural flow of feelings and eventually the ability to grieve. Children may not be in touch with their feelings of grief, or those feelings may be ambivalent and in conflict with each other. A sudden or traumatic loss poses a higher risk for complicated grief.

DEVELOPMENTAL ASPECTS IN THE GRIEF PROCESS

The question "Can children mourn?" has been asked and debated in the literature. Webb (2002a) suggests that the significant reactions of preschool children to the loss of a meaningful person may qualify as "grief reactions" rather than as "mourning," because these children lack the understanding of the finality or meaning of that loss. With respect to schoolchildren, developmental stages must be carefully considered. Schoolchildren possess sufficient understanding of the finality of death, which usually develops around age six. However, the meaning of the loss of a significant adult to children changes at different ages. What children experience as stressful will also differ depending on their developmental stage.

At the age of 6, children see the parent primarily as someone who does things to meet their needs (Silverman, 2000). At 8 years old, children begin to be aware of their needs for someone who will not only do things for them but also with them, and children can now articulate that the parent should provide them with security or certainty. As children mature further, they can realize that what is lost is the developing interaction with the deceased parent. They can now set aside their own needs and be aware of the other person in his or her own right (Silverman, 2000). School age children up to the age of 9 may disavow death and utilize denial as a defense mechanism and may thus appear unaffected. Although by this age children usually understand the reality of death in terms of its irreversibility, they may continue to believe it can only happen to other people and that thoughts can cause accidents and death to happen. Although they encounter strong feelings of loss, children may often find it difficult to express these emotions; they are often unprepared for the length of the grieving process and may thus deny their grief. They may have one or more of the following symptoms: eating and sleeping difficulties, headaches and stomachaches, excessive fearfulness, guilt feelings, anger directed at certain people who they perceive allowed or even "caused" the death (e.g., God, doctors, a parent). Anger may be directed toward a teacher or a classmate. Classroom behavior may become inappropriate, concentration may weaken, and school performance may decline.

From preadolescence through adolescence, children gain a progressively more mature view of death and understand its universality, irreversibility, permanence, and (personal) mortality. Adolescents' adult-like stance with respect to death is mediated by tensions unique to this period in life (Noppe & Noppe, 1996). During latency, talking about painful events remains difficult, and children are capable of depressive symptomatology (and even suicidal ideation). By puberty, youngsters tend to become more egocentric, and, thus, most are inclined to be preoccupied with how the death affects them personally; they give less (or no) consideration to its impact on others. As the struggle to assert independence (especially emotional separation from parents) becomes increasingly important, it may be shocking for the child to realize the enormity of the loss of a parent and how needed the deceased was.

Adolescents' omnipotence may serve as a counter phobic reaction to the fear of the reality of death; they may still view themselves as immortal. Teenagers may romanticize death (e.g., death by suicide), be attracted to spiritualistic beliefs, and become excessively preoccupied with ideas regarding "the meaning of life," what happens after death, and the purpose of life. A shattering of life assumptions (Janoff-Bulman, 1985, 1992) can lead to philosophical questions, mood swings, and depression (Gudas, 1993). In addition to symptoms seen in younger children, adolescents' symptomatology may also reveal a lack of energy and eating disorders. They may respond, too, with risk-taking behaviors such as self-medication via drugs and alcohol or involvement in sexual promiscuity.

Beyond the aforesaid common age-group responses, some gender differences in the adjustment process have been reported as well. Generally, males behave more aggressively; they may test authority figures and (especially adolescents) are likely to abuse drugs and alcohol. In contrast, females tend to reach out more for support and consolation (Fleming & Balmer, 1996; Raphael, 1983). It should be acknowledged, however, that individual children's responses are not merely a function of their gender, age, and stage of development. Biology and culture, and the specific recovery environment, working together, may account for both commonalties and differences in children's response to loss.

TRAUMATIC LOSS

Although all deaths may be perceived as personally traumatic, some circumstances are objectively traumatic (Rando, 1993). These objective circumstances involve the death's sudden timing, violent or cruel cause, randomness, and/or multiplicity (e.g., death of both parents). A sudden, unexpected loss that contradicts the normal expectable life trajectory may be particularly devastating in itself because the bereaved has no time for emotional preparation and little (if any) time to make cognitive and intrapersonal adjustments. Add to the unexpectedness other factors such as violence or multiple deaths, and the result may be bereavement overload that places the child at risk for adjustment problems. Death caused by disaster thus deserves special consideration as a *traumatic loss*, involving elements of sudden, perhaps horrific, shocking encounters *in addition* to the loss of a loved one (Raphael, 1997).

The terms *traumatic death, traumatic grief, traumatic bereavement, and complicated grief* are often used interchangeably (Prigerson et al., 1997). It may be argued, however, that traumatic grief or bereavement constitutes a separate conceptual entity that should be restricted to losses in events that would independently be classified as trauma, irrespective of the response or the interpretation of the particular bereaved individual (Rubin, Malkinson, & Witztum, 2000). Traumatic grief/bereavement increases the risk for complicated (prolonged, difficult, exaggerated, distorted, or blocked) grief; nonetheless, complicated grief/bereavement does not result exclusively from traumatic death.

Traumatic grief/bereavement involves a complex overlay of symptoms that arise from a difficulty in moving on with the grief processes due to a preoccupation with the trauma, thereby impairing "normal" grief work. For instance, bereaved persons who witnessed a violent death may continue to be preoccupied by images from the violent event and by emotional reactions of acute pangs of helplessness (Brom & Kleber, 2000). Without first working through the traumatic experience or the traumatic nature of the death, these additional difficulties may impede normal grief work and resolution (Nader, 1997). Nader described, for example, a second grader who, after a tornado, was unable to focus upon issues of grief until she reenacted her experience of a wall collapsing and her dead sister's inaction prior to her death. The girl remained emotionally flat until she was assisted to express her anger at her sister for not running to safety. Only then did she become animated, could continue the story of her traumatic experience, and was able to begin to enact elements of her grief experience.

Elementary school students who endured a sniper attack on their school playground were at times observed to manifest grief independently from traumatic stress, whereas at other times these reactions appeared to be in interplay with one another (Pynoos et al., 1987). Loss and trauma can thus be seen as separate but sometimes-related entities. In both processes, reexperiencing and preoccupation dominate, but each expresses different specific contents. The dominant features of traumatic reactions comprise intrusion and preoccupation with traumatic content, whereas bereavement's dominant content involves preoccupation with the lost person. Arousal and avoidance play an essential part in the clinical picture for traumatic reactions but are less pronounced in bereavement. With regard to pathways to disorder, the sequelae of traumatic reactions may lead to PTSD, but the sequelae of bereavement reactions usually center on types of complicated grief and depression (Rubin et al., 2000). Similarities do exist between the processing of traumatic events and the processing of traumatic loss, but these relate more to the form of the coping process than to its content. Contents may differ widely; yet, coping patterns and the factors influencing the coping process are similar (Brom & Kleber, 2000).

In general, the combination of trauma and bereavement may result in prolonged symptoms (McCann & Pearlman, 1990). Traumatic death is associated with a higher risk for persistent forms of grief. In many cases, traumatic loss may require more time to process than do other forms of loss. School-age children may be particularly vulnerable to the dual demands of trauma mastery and grief work (Pynoos & Nader, 1988). Unsuccessful attempts at trauma processing can complicate the bereavement process and increase the likelihood of traumatic grief. Thus, intervention for relieving trauma-associated anxiety should take psychological priority over mourning.

A disaster that does not involve the death of a loved one may require less actual adaptation in behavioral and interaction patterns than when the death of a loved one is involved. Bereaved trauma survivors report higher levels of PTSD symptoms compared to trauma survivors who did not also experience the death of a loved one. In the Oklahoma City bombing, children who lost a friend experienced significantly more PTSD symptoms than those who lost an acquaintance, and children who lost an immediate family member experienced significantly more symptoms than did any other survivors (Pfefferbaum et al., 1999).

THE SECONDARY EFFECTS OF TRAUMATIC DEATH

Traumatic death may often result in an unstable environment for the child. Both clinical and empirical studies emphasize that it is the presence of a secure relationship with a trusted adult who provides consistency, comfort, and prompt and accurate age-appropriate information that helps in processing grief successfully (Gudas, 1993). However, children exposed to both death and disaster may be denied the availability of a supporting adult. (See the following chapter for an elaboration on the effect of traumatic events on the family.) Surviving adults often evidence difficulties of their own both in responding to the impact of the disaster itself and in dealing with their own grief. Consequently, adults may be unresponsive or even unaware of the loss's psychological impact on the child. Furthermore, the psychological availability and support of siblings may diminish concurrently, when they employ avoidant defense mechanisms or become emotionally disengaged from the grieving family. The family's habitual mode of organizing and relating thus undergoes dramatic alterations that affect the parenting and sibling subsystems as well as the sense of security and stability in the child's emotional and actual everyday life.

Moreover, the often-chaotic circumstances surrounding the disaster may generate disaster-specific barriers to environmental support for children's bereavement and trauma processing. Investment of extraordinary efforts into rescue and recovery may result in the grief being neither openly acknowledged nor publicly mourned for some time. Especially when disasters involve multiple losses of significant others, children may develop intense insecurity and fear of abandonment. Confusion over the circumstances of death, inability to recover the body, or failure to identify the body of the deceased person may arouse additional anxieties. When the body of the deceased cannot be found, survivors may contrive elaborate explanations to convince themselves that their loved ones are still alive but elsewhere (Cohen, 1987). These additional disaster-specific difficulties may interact with other difficulties that are not necessarily disaster-related. Such difficulties in the grief process include the chasm created in the lives of family members (e. g., lack of role model), an ambivalent relationship to the deceased that may result in over-exaggeration of one characteristic response (e.g., guilt, anger), or social stigma associated with the death (e.g., when it is embarrassing to speak of the deceased's behavior).

In cases of an unstable postdisaster environment, children may become particularly confused and disturbed by their normal grief reactions and thus refrain from manifestations of sadness and other intense reactions. Caretakers must attend to this possibility and make an effort to help children with reassurance and support when needed.

Chapter 7

The Effects of Traumatic Events on the Family, the Parent-Child Relationship, and the Parent-School Partnership

In this chapter, we attempt to highlight the importance of viewing the child's responses to trauma within the context of family relationships and family-school relationships. To clarify children's needs and design effective school-based interventions with families, intervention planners must understand the multiplicity of relationships and the complex interpersonal processes that mediate children's adjustment.

EFFECTS OF TRAUMA ON THE FAMILY

The impact of traumatic events is never confined solely to an affected individual. It inevitably impinges, both directly and indirectly, on the lives of the child's family and significant others in various ways. In events that directly involve the whole family, each member is faced with the double challenge of processing his or her subjective traumatic experience and managing individual reactions, while concurrently being aware of and reacting to the experiences of the others. A major notion of the family system approach depicts the "interconnectedness" of family members, implying that even in incidents exposing only a single family member to a traumatic event, the entire family system will be immediately and often dramatically affected. Members of the family tend to identify with the affected family member, to share the traumatic experience and its impact through their intimate psychological ties with that individual, and thus may endure a *secondary traumatization* as well as the *contagious effect* of posttraumatic reactions (Steinberg, 1998). For example, some or all family members may show increased arousal and hypervigilance, avoidance of trauma reminders, or distress at exposure to cues symbolizing the event, even if they were not the family members directly exposed to it.

Siblings of children who were victims of violence or disaster stand at risk for developing various emotional difficulties, including PTSD (Newman, Black, & Harris-Hendriks, 1997). The little research conducted on parents' mechanisms of secondary traumatization (Barnes, 1998) suggests that under extreme circumstances, parents can be pushed beyond their "stress absorption" capacity, and when that point is passed the development of young children can deteriorate rapidly and markedly (Garbarino, 1995). Changes in the functional level of stressed parents may not only evoke a chain of emotional reactions, but also confront the family with new practical demands and adaptations that may themselves become a source of serious stress. For example, when soldiers are deployed overseas, such as occurred during the Vietnam War or the Gulf War, the remaining family members need to cope both with anxiety about the welfare of their loved one on the front lines, and with the added responsibilities stemming from the soldier's absence in the everyday operation of the household. The remaining parent may become much less available to tend to children's needs under such circumstances. Children may be pushed into premature independence and self-sufficiency, which may prove to be beyond their coping capacity.

This combination of both increased functional demands and emotional stress especially manifests itself in families with additional postdisaster stressors or where one parent develops PTSD, such as the case of returning war veterans. Additional family stressors, such as death or hospitalization of a significant adult or parental divorce or separation, appear to impede recovery and predict PTSD symptoms in children over time (Silverman & La Greca, 2002). The literature on war veterans affected by PTSD indicates that their guilt feelings, emotional withdrawal, and elevated levels of aggression make it difficult, perhaps even impossible, for veterans to fully resume their former roles of parent, spouse, and wage earner. Furthermore, spouses and children of these veterans revealed a high incidence of stress reactions and psychopathological symptoms (Arzi, Solomon, & Dekel, 2000; Solomon, 1988), even though they were not directly exposed to the war-related traumatizing experiences. These familial reactions may be attributed both to secondary traumatization as well as to the difficulty in adapting to the added emotional demands and new functional burden involved in living with a disabled PTSD spouse or parent. Often, when PTSD severely disables one parent and the other parent exhibits reactive symptoms in the face of the new and stressful family situation, children may experience not only secondary traumatization but also the loss of parental availability and support from both parents.

THE LINK BETWEEN FAMILY FUNCTIONING AND CHILDREN'S ADAPTATION FOLLOWING A TRAUMATIC EVENT

Parental emotional reactions to a traumatic event constitute a powerful mediator of the child"s posttraumatic symptoms (AACAP, 1998). Two comprehensive reviews of the relevant literature yielded consistent evidence supporting this claim. Scheeringa and Zeanah (2001) reviewed 17 studies that simultaneously assessed parental and child functioning following trauma, and Norris et al. (2002a) summarized the research from 19 samples regarding the influence of family factors on child outcomes following trauma. The emergent picture from both reviews shows a clear pattern of relational links between parental functioning and child functioning, following disasters and traumatic events. The parental and family variables that emerged as associated with the poorest child outcomes included: higher rates of PTSD in either parent; parents' higher rates of posttraumatic symptoms, anxieties, and psychiatric problems; increased parental conflict and irritability; family chaos; and inadequate family cohesion. Specific parental behaviors conspicuous in their negative impact on the parent-child dynamics and the child's adjustment included mother's avoidance of the trauma, parental suppression of awareness about their child's symptoms, and parental behaviors that induced guilt and anxiety in the child. The importance of an adequate, supportive relational context for children's ability to process a traumatic event is further amplified during events involving the loss of a family member. As described in Chapter 6, for the surviving child, the loss of one parent, or of a sibling, often becomes a multiple loss experience. The bereaved child may feel deprived not only of the deceased, but also of the much-needed sustaining relationship with the surviving parent, who is often psychologically unavailable due to his or her own grief. Likewise, the psychological availability and support of siblings may diminish concurrently.

Even in instances where the child is the victim of a traumatic event (either via direct exposure or proximity to a victim), parents vary in their ability to provide the child with the attuned, sensitive, and supportive parenting that the child needs. We have observed that parents' initial reactions upon learning of the child's plight often involve alarm and panic reactions, confusion, and a sense of helplessness. Extreme parental behavior may emerge in the form of either paralysis or excessive overprotectiveness and agitation. The sources of these reactions are manifold. Many parents find it especially difficult to regulate their own affective reactions to the actual or perceived threat to their own child's life. In line with Stern's (1995) description of the way parents psychologically organize their parenting role ("the motherhood constellation"), this threat may symbolize a frightening, painful, and guilt evoking failure in their capacity to protect their child from harm. This loss of self-confidence in the ability to fulfill the major parental role, namely, to sustain and safeguard one's child's life, may be further amplified by the parent's lack of knowledge and skills in the area of coping with the child's trauma and posttraumatic reactions. The child's reactions can be unfamiliar to the parents, who may feel that their child has been altered by the unusual event, and consequently even fear that the event caused the child psychological and developmental damage. The parent's fear of causing further harm to the child by inappropriately reacting to or handling the child's behavior may further aggravate the parent's sense of demobilization and incapacitation. Furthermore, parents often feel ill equipped to explain to their children the occurrence of such cruel and often extremely inhumane events as those evidenced in violent deliberate human acts. They may also find themselves unable to withstand the emotional pain of the child's shattered illusions.

At these times, shortly after the acute impact phase, parents may expect specialists at the school or hospital to "take over" and brief and debrief the child, tell the child the bad news, or even treat the child to "erase the marks of trauma." Alternatively, some parents' use of denial and avoidance as defense mechanisms to deal with their own anxieties and guilt may preclude their recognition of children's signs of distress. A number of studies have documented this pattern of denial, showing meaningful discrepancies between children's self-reports of posttraumatic stress reactions and their parents' reports (Barnes, 1998; Salmon & Bryant, 2002; Scheeringa & Zeanah, 2001).

Implications for Intervention

The significant role of family dynamics, and especially the parenting process, in the child's adjustment during the aftermath of a traumatic event holds important implications for intervention. We believe that parents constitute a major resource for children's coping and should be proactively helped to remain so, even when their parenting capacities are threatened or temporarily diminished by trauma. Family-centered interventions should therefore be designed to empower parents at these critical times, so they can provide, at least partially, a "healing" context for their children. This coincides with the U.S. National Institute of Mental Health recommendations (2003) stating that the family should be considered the first-line resource for helping children deal with a catastrophe, to promote a faster and better adjustment. Interventions with parents around disasters may thus involve a double focus: parents as affected individuals and parents as helpers. As adults affected by the trauma, and especially when traumatized themselves, parents may need support in regulating their own emotions and in handling their own confusion and neediness. Norris and her collaborators (2002a, 2002b) maintained that provision of care and support to stressed parents can most effectively furnish care and support to the children affected by disaster. In Chapter 13, we detail a system of school-based preventive interventions with parents to meet these objectives.

Additionally, at these times, most parents need education and training with regard to their role vis-à-vis their children, and the majority expect inputs from professionals as to how best to help their child work through this unusual ordeal. Therefore, trauma work should carefully avoid the traditional division between mental health services for adults and for children and, instead, should allow for integrative flexible services of a consultative or therapeutic nature for both sets of clients.

Mechanisms of Parental Influence

To clarify more fully the mechanisms by which parents affect their children's adjustment and maladjustment in adverse situations, we will next draw on the large body of research findings that link the quality of child adjustment following traumatic events to parent-child experiences. Understanding these mechanisms will then enable the consideration of central implications for interventions designed to help parents help their children. Parental contributions to children's coping with disaster can be conceptualized as involving four main mechanisms: attachment ties and processes; signaling, interpreting, and modeling; processing feelings and thoughts and correcting misconceptions; and relational patterns between parent and child.

Attachment Ties and Processes

Bowlby (1969) emphasized that attachment behavior is first of all a vital biological function, indispensable for both reproduction and survival. A rapidly expanding body of research has shown that disturbances of childhood attachment bonds can render long-term neurobiological consequences. Beyond disturbances in affect regulation, a large variety of both human and animal research has shown that childhood abuse, neglect, and separation cause far-reaching biopsychosocial effects. Such effects include lasting biological changes that affect the capacity to modulate emotions, difficulty in learning new coping skills, and impairment in the capacity to engage in meaningful social affiliations (Schore, 2001).

Based on predictions from attachment theory, a number of studies demonstrated that children who formed secure attachments to their parents, and those who came from more stable families, did demonstrate greater resilience following traumatic events (Bowlby, 1988; Luthar & Zigler, 1991; Wright et al., 1997). Several mechanisms, which are not mutually exclusive, may explicate these findings. First, stable and nurturing families appear to provide children with *inner resources* that enhance coping ability and serve as a protective shield when the children are confronted with a traumatic event. These resources, according to attachment theory, may include optimism, self-reliance, a sense of self-worth, trust in others, and the ability to use relationships and to cooperate with others (Egeland, Carlson, & Sroufe, 1993). Second, these families are better able to provide the child with adequate *immediate and sustaining support*, and to effectively *organize their child's environment* when disaster strikes. These secure parents continue to protect the children's sense of stability, permanence, and competence, thus helping their children to retain a strong positive attachment to their families and to cope better with the stress of the traumatic events (Garbarino, 1992). These parents also appear much more *attentive* to the children's signs of distress than do distressed parents, and are more *available to soothe and support* children in stressful times (La Greca, 2001).

When a traumatic event disrupts the child's sense of security and predictability about the world and shatters the child's "basic assumptions" (Janoff-Bulman, 1992), the child's *attachment system* is activated, including the need to establish a *secure base* by reuniting with significant caretakers (Gordon, Farberow, & Maida, 1999; Scheeringa & Zeanah, 2001). The functions of the family as an important attachment system are exemplified in studies showing the harmful effects of forced separation from family members, chiefly in traumatic times. Traumatized children and youth who were separated from their nuclear family, whether in Cambodia, Yugoslavia, or Israel (Kinzie, Sack, Angell, Manson, & Rath, 1986; Lahad, Shacham & Niv, 2000), exhibited greater behavioral difficulties and poorer long-term adjustment in comparison with those who were not separated or who quickly rejoined members of their families. Children who were reunited together with even one member of the nuclear family adjusted better than those who remained separated entirely from their families.

However, the mere physical presence of a parent does not suffice to ensure that a child will receive desperately needed emotional support from attachment figures during confusing, stressful times. Substantial evidence regarding the correlation between parental and child distress and symptomatology (Benedek, 1985; Breton, Valla, & Lambert, 1993; Harkness, 1993) suggests that distressed parents are often less available emotionally to support their children in comparison with parents who show adaptive psychological functioning in times of crisis.

Certainly, the psychological rather than physical availability of parents constitutes the factor of consequence. Parents who can regulate their own emotions, actually listen to the child's concerns, reaffirm their love and protection, help regulate the child's emotions, and solve problems offer their children a truly supportive, "holding" environment conducive to children's recovery from trauma.

Signaling, Interpreting, and Modeling

In unusual times such as war, emergency, or disaster, the parents' conduct and reactions appear to serve a central function in social signaling and referencing for their children. Like adults, children need to reconstruct a sense of continuity following disaster. Inasmuch as children are less familiar and less experienced than adults with the new complex world created by unexpected events, they rely on adults' appraisals of the traumatic situation. Thus, children use their parents' behavior to construe the meaning and significance of events and to evaluate the severity of existing or potential risk. In reality, children often seem to react more to their parents' expressions of distress than to the distressing events per se. Younger children rely more heavily on parental stress responses as cues for interpreting traumatic events, in comparison to older children. It is helpful to children when adults are able to communicate to them that the situation, or part of it, is under control, that the child's response is appropriate under such unusual circumstances, and that the parents are coping and are confident that things will improve (Klingman, 2001b).

In a study of stress and coping reactions among Israeli children under the threat of Scud missile attacks during the Gulf war, parents' negative reactions correlated positively with children's level of emotional distress and with children's frequency of somatic complaints and everyday difficulties (Bat-Zion & Levy-Shiff, 1993). In contrast, *expressions of positive emotions* by parents correlated with children's positive coping.

Further support for the *interpretative-evaluative function* that parental reactions serve for children in unusual circumstances can be gained from a study examining the mediating effect of parents' reactions to television reports that cover stressful events, on children's reactions. In this study, a strong association emerged between the attitudes and the emotional reactions of Dutch, British, and American children who were not directly exposed to any war, and the attitudes expressed by their parents following television reports on the Gulf War (Greenberg, 1993).

Parents' actual coping behavior probably also conveys significant communication to children about safety and optimism. Shahinfar and Fox (1997) have suggested that parents who themselves deal effectively with a traumatic situation thereby *model* appropriate coping strategies for their children. Parents' responses to their children's behavior also directly communicate their evaluative stance. These responses, when delivered contingently, play a strong role in decreasing or increasing targeted child behaviors. Parents may thus influence their children's coping behavior unintentionally. Researchers have shown that parents of anxious children reinforce their children's avoidant behavior more than do parents of non-anxious children, who seem to encourage active coping (Salmon & Bryant, 2002).

Parents may *reinforce desired behaviors* by providing positive attention and approval and by gradually *shaping* the child's coping strategies. For example, the use of planned shaping and positive reinforcements by parents increased young children's cooperation in wearing a gas mask during the Gulf War (Klingman, 1992).

Processing Feelings and Thoughts, and Correcting Misconceptions

Children need help in making sense out of their traumatic experience and in integrating it into their existing schemas. Salmon and Bryant (2002) documented the contribution of parents' willingness and *ability to converse* with their children concerning the traumatic experience. These authors emphasized the contribution of these conversations to language development and narrative production in the child, which comprise necessary elements of *trauma processing*. Because negative emotions are more difficult to process and more anxiety provoking, children seem to benefit from the help of parents who actively relate to their children's negative emotions.

It seems that parents who are too distressed themselves, or those who try to shield their child from the negative impact of trauma, tend to avoid talking about the experience with their children. Parents' avoidant behavior may thus deprive the child of opportunities to *reappraise the experience and correct misconceptions*, as well as to *regulate strong emotions*. Parental avoidance may also explain the findings of Laor, Wolmer, Mayes, and Gershon (1997), who conducted a follow-up study of Israeli preschoolers displaced from their homes as a result of Scud missile attacks. Whereas most children recovered from their stress symptoms rather quickly, those children who remained symptomatic were more likely to have mothers who were exhibiting avoidant symptoms. This avoidance may account for the children's difficulty in successfully processing the trauma like their peers. Other studies have also shown an association between mother's avoidance of trauma-related material and an increase in her child's posttraumatic symptoms (Laor et al., 1997; Pynoos, Steinberg, & Goenjian, 1996; Scheeringa & Zeanah, 2001).

RELATIONAL PATTERNS BETWEEN PARENT AND CHILD

It is important to keep in mind that the influences of parents on children, however, are not unidirectional. All participants in intimate interactions contribute to the construction of a unique pattern of relating and communicating. The mutual or separate trauma experiences in the family may alter patterns of relating in a number of rather predictable ways. Thus, not only may parents become insecure about their ability to protect their children, but also the traumatized child may lose faith in the efficacy and power of the parents (Pynoos et al., 1996). To defend against this frightening realization, the child may engage in developmentally inappropriate behaviors like extreme clinginess and dependency or, conversely, premature independence and self-reliance. Indeed, children living under conditions of violence and war have been described as "growing up too soon," a development predicted to result in negative psychological consequences (Punamaki, Qouta, & El Sarraj, 1997). Parents may misinterpret these changes. Not realizing that it serves as a defense mechanism, parents may become supportive and proud of a child's new, seemingly self-reliant and daring behavior. Alternatively, they may overprotect a clingy child in response to their own anxiety, and thus inadvertently validate the child's anxiety and sense that, indeed, protection is needed.

Punamaki et al.'s (1997) findings are of particular interest in demonstrating the complexity of the changes in relational patterns between children and parents. They reported that in Palestinian families exposed to events involving violence, loss, and destruction, as children experienced more traumatic events, they perceived their parents to be more punishing, rejecting, and controlling. Although the data in the study derived solely from children's reports, it is reasonable to assume that these perceptions reflected both actual changes in parental behaviors as a result of the familial stress, as well as feelings projected onto the parental figures by the stressed children. These perceptions, however, must have strongly affected the parent-child relationship and contributed to child behavior problems.

Scheeringa and Zeanah (2001) observed three problematic relational patterns that tend to emerge as the result of the co-concurrence of posttraumatic reactions in an adult caregiver and a young child. One parenting pattern involves adult withdrawal and diminished availability and responsiveness toward the child. This pattern may be related to a previous trauma or loss suffered by the parent, which is reawakened by the child's trauma. A second parenting pattern, which is probably more common, involves overprotecting the child and using rigid unwarranted restrictions of the child's actions, possibly in a defensive attempt to rectify the sense of loss of control and guilt evoked by the child's exposure to the trauma. This pattern is similar to the one observed in Palestinian mothers who tended to compensate their children for their suffering in traumatic times (Punamaki et al., 1997). The third parenting pattern suggested by Scheeringa and Zeanah is most worrisome. This pattern refers to adult acts of reenacting, endangering, and frightening the young child, due to an excessive, relentless preoccupation with the trauma. In such cases, the adult's traumatic needs take precedence, and the child's needs are ignored. It appears that adult loneliness may contribute to the consolidation of this pattern. Scheeringa and Zeanah pointed out that any of these three parental responses might complicate or impede children's recovery. These authors suggested the introduction of dyadic therapeutic interventions in such cases, where the parent interacts with the child (usually in play) in the presence of a therapist. The therapist intervenes to help the parent become more attuned to the child's experience and communications and to respond more sensitively. Scheeringa and Zeanah accentuated the parental role in instigating these three relational patterns, but the young child, too, may contribute and help shape these patterns. Children's depression, anxieties, and PTSD reactions may feed into each of the aforementioned patterns.

Two additional common patterns, which we have observed in our clinical work with families bereaved by the Yom Kippur War, comprise psychological role reversal and child scapegoating. These patterns tend to emerge especially in cases where parents are gravely affected by the trauma and lack sufficient psychosocial resources. Role reversal reflects children's tendency to assume adult roles when traumatic circumstances (e.g., political violence) do not allow parents to protect the children, forcing children to grow up too soon (Punamaki et. al., 1997). Children who collaborate in the role-reversal pattern are often sensitive and mature in their social capabilities. They assume the role of caretaker: They worry about the parent's mood, become vigilant about the parent's safety, avoid burdening the parent with their own issues, and attempt to encourage and please the parent. These efforts may be accompanied by anxiety and guilt, as this assumed new role places a serious burden on the child, which is inappropriate for the child's developmental capabilities and tasks.

Scapegoating consists of an even more problematic pattern that occurs when the child internalizes the negative and angry feelings that are communicated to the child, either indiscriminately or directly, by a traumatized and out-of-control parent. The parent's rejecting or blaming reactions evoke acting-up behavior in the child, who thus assumes the role of someone "evil" who is considered responsible for the parent's frustration, anger, and sadness. Such a process of child scapegoating in the family enables both parent and child to avoid dealing with the issues of trauma by focusing instead on their intense relational conflict. However, this pattern sets in motion a cycle of destructive unresolved behavior problems. Hobfoll and his colleagues (Hobfoll et al., 1991) reported that families exposed to war may show symptoms such as physical violence and scapegoating of the children for family difficulties.

Cases of parental withdrawal, over-protectiveness, endangerment, role reversal, or scapegoating call for systemic family interventions as well as individual therapy for parents, rather than child therapy. Attachment theory and research as well as clinical case reports concur that treatment of the parent is critical for child recovery in such cases, especially when children are young (see Scheeringa & Zeanah, 2001). In less extreme cases, the emotional toll of parenting in times of trauma necessitates a support system for parents and for children, which can be developed through the school system.

RELATIONAL PATTERNS BETWEEN PARENTS AND SCHOOLS

Children's adjustment following a traumatic event may reflect their relationship with their parents as well as with their school, and also be influenced by the quality of their parents' relationship with the school.

Schools may potentially serve as an additional *secure base* for children when family resources are limited. The school can provide a sense of security through its stability of relationships with significant others (e.g., teachers and peers); its routines, activities, and structures; and its formal and informal opportunities to communicate, share, express feelings, and raise questions concerning upsetting events. Teachers who are attentive to their students may play a supportive role for parents, helping to alleviate parents' excessive worries about their children by keeping them informed about the child's functioning at school and about the classroom activities related to the traumatic material. When necessary, teachers may also sensitize the parents to changes in their child's behavior. Often, however, teachers use avoidance and denial to cope with their own anxieties. They may try to overprotect parents, especially if the family has suffered a loss, or if the parents appear extremely stressed. When speaking to parents, teachers may try to conceal or play down worrisome changes in a child's functioning. At other times, teachers may feel angry and resentful towards parents, especially when they are perceived as being preoccupied and neglectful of the child's needs. Teachers themselves require support and guidance from a school mental health consultant to work out their own feelings and learn how to sensitively and effectively approach parents. The possible hazards of denial and avoidance in dealing with difficult memories and feelings must be addressed in the training of teachers.

Schools may also become a support system for the parents themselves, by organizing a range of supportive activities and interventions that are designed to address specific parental needs at different stages of coping with the trauma (see Chapter 13). Relevant personnel, who have been previously trained in crisis intervention, can conduct these interventions and, when needed, call on the support of crisis teams from the area or from collaborating mental health agencies.

Our work in the schools over the years has taught us that prior investment in parent-school relationships will substantially determine the school's ability to enlist parents both as partners and as clients in times of crisis. One such crisis was experienced by a Tel Aviv high school after a group of its students were tragically killed by a suicide-bomb attack at a discotheque over the weekend (in June 2001). The principal attributed the students' successful coping with this disaster to the preexisting warm and caring relationships between school staff and families (A. Benbenishti, personal communication, December 18, 2002). In the aftermath of the tragedy, the school continued to view the affected families, all relatively new immigrants from Russia, as part of the school community. The principle took responsibility for tending to their material and emotional needs, such as helping to organize the funerals and encouraging students to continue their visits with the bereaved families after the initial mourning period.

Familiarity with the school population's characteristics, the families' strengths and vulnerabilities, and the community's organization and resources contribute immeasurably to school-based interventions around trauma. Such familiarity may facilitate decisions on priorities for intervention, guide the organization of self-help activities within the school population, and foster the identification of high-risk children. Prior connections with various religious leaders and organizations with which the families in a particular school are involved, for example, may provide a tremendous resource when planning appropriate participation and respectful support for bereaved students and families.

As people under hardship often pull together, join ranks, and experience a sense of communality (Breznitz, 1983), it may also be argued that a crisis situation presents a new opportunity for the school and parents to rebuild a fragile relationship. However, this may not be a simple undertaking when both parties feel needy and insecure and are confronting such unusual circumstances. One should be cognizant of the fact that traumatic events may also aggravate any existing problematic relationships between schools and parents. The anxieties and tension evoked by the trauma may make trusting one another a difficult endeavor for all involved. Parents may become suspicious, challenge the school's policies, and question its ability to protect the children from harm. Families may doubt the ability of school personnel to deal with the processing of children's traumatic experiences. Parents may even withdraw the child from school, or convey a message of mistrust to the child about the school, thus compromising the child's sense of security and inadvertently encouraging such reactions as school refusal or behavior problems in the classroom. Similar parental messages targeted at specific teachers can aggravate the blow to teachers' sense of self-efficacy, which may already be quite shaken as a result of the traumatic event.

A typical compensatory reaction to the perceived lack of control related to the trauma involves the tendency of either parents or school personnel to exercise more rigid control over postdisaster decision-making issues. This tendency manifests itself especially around such issues as safety, psychological handling of the trauma, memorializing, and returning to routine. Family privacy and autonomy may be argued as justification for inhibiting the school's proactive actions around issues of trauma. Parent-school relations may thereby take the form of a power struggle rather than a collaborative problem-solving effort. A case in point relates to the parental demand for control evidenced in one New York City school affected by the WTC disaster (Personal communication by anonymous parents, November, 2001). At a parent assembly meeting following the resumption of school, a number of parents demanded that teachers be forbidden from talking to their students about their shared and vivid traumatic experience and, further, that students be forbidden from speaking to one another about their experiences.

Conversely, parents may express very high expectations toward the school, hoping that the institution will take over where they feel confused and helpless. In a Jerusalem school following a terrorist bus explosion, for example, parents asked if school personnel could notify their child about the loss of a family relative, hoping to avoid having to be the informants (Personal communication by an anonymous school psychologist, October, 2002). In both of these examples, to help avoid engagement in conflict with these parents, school personnel should try to understand the dynamics at play – of anxiety and the sense of loss of control or competence – that fuel such parental requests. By addressing parental concerns in an accepting manner and by offering guidance such as expert information on the importance of processing trauma (with the coordinated help of natural support systems), school personnel may play a vital role in defusing debilitating or unhelpful reactive patterns.

Disaster also provides an opportunity for those people involved in caring for children to pull together and establish a more dedicated, collaborative, and resourceful community, equipped to deal with the children's difficulties. For example, in various schools in Israel, parents' meetings were held together with school personnel in the wake of the outbreak of terrorist acts in late 2001 due to the Palestinian uprising. These meetings revealed a common concern about children's safety in the afternoons, while playing in unsupervised neighborhood parks, yards, and playgrounds. The mutual discussion of this problem was instrumental in initiating supervised afterschool programs in the community, designed in response to parents' concerns.

Chapter 8

Coping, Habituation, Resilience, and Trauma-Induced Growth

I n the previous chapters of this book, we have outlined various negative impacts of community disaster as it renders stress, trauma, and bereavement on survivors. Yet, as we described in our core assumptions in the first section of the book, we do not view disasters as simply impinging on schoolchildren who are passive recipients of environmental forces. The impact of disasters on children and adolescents will vary as a function of their resources and their efforts at processing the disaster-related effects. Indeed, many people adjust well to disaster despite exposure to extremely stressful circumstances. Some children mature more rapidly after having managed stressful events effectively. Some report being positively changed, in the longer run, by their struggle with trauma. The study of children in war and warlike zones has led to understanding that, often, exposure to repeated and increased stress doses builds up protective mechanisms, and that children in particularly difficult circumstances can learn to cope better (Aptekar & Stoecklin, 1997). In this section of the book, we will introduce these empowering, positive resources. We will review the psychological theories and research findings about coping, resiliency, and growth related to disaster and trauma, and we will discuss their implications for intervention.

COPING AND ADJUSTMENT

It is now commonly recognized that stress per se does not determine adaptive outcomes, but rather *how we cope* with stress comprises the crucial factor. When individuals perceive their coping resources as sufficient to meet their environmental and inner (emotional) demands, they appraise the stressful situation as less threatening and may even consider it challenging. Coping involves the person's constantly changing emotional, cognitive, and behavioral efforts undertaken to manage, master, tolerate, or minimize specific external (environmental) and/or internal (intrapsychic) demands that the person perceives as representing potential threats, existing harms, or losses, and as taxing or exceeding the person's existing resources (Folkman & Lazarus, 1985).

Researchers have identified two broad categories or types of coping: problem-focused and emotion-focused (Lazarus & Folkman, 1984). *Problem-focused coping* involves direct efforts aimed at doing something to alter the source of the stress. *Emotion-focused coping* comprises efforts aimed at reducing or managing the emotional distress associated with the problem or the situation. Problem-focused skills appear to be acquired earlier, probably because many of these skills involve overt behaviors that are easily observed even by young children, and tend to be more readily acquired through modeling of adult behaviors. Younger children have less access to their own internal emotional states, and often fail to recognize that their emotions can be brought under self-regulation.

Coping may also be characterized with respect to its approach versus avoidant mode and with respect to its cognitive or behavioral method (Moos, 2002). *Cognitive approaching coping* would include positive appraisal as well as logical analysis (e.g., drawing on past experiences, going over the new situation in one's mind to try to understand it). *Cognitive avoidant coping* connotes escapism, inattention, repression ("forgetting the whole thing"), or attempts to evade any thoughts or reminders of the disastrous event, thus reducing arousal and intrusions. Avoidance may enable the person to approach the trauma-induced emotions and cognitions gradually, in small doses, without becoming overwhelmed by them (Ginzburg, Solomon, & Bleich, 2002). Problem solving, designing and following a plan of action, and actively seeking support reflect *behavioral approaching coping*. Intended withdrawal and the pursuit of alternative rewards that require active engagement and enable emotional discharge exemplify *behavioral avoidant coping*.

The transactional approach to coping, which is the most prevalent, views coping as constantly changing, emphasizes the role of situation appraisal as central to the choice of strategy, and acknowledges human flexibility in choosing coping strategies. Adaptive coping may differ across types of disasters and at different points in the course of a disastrous episode (Compas & Epping, 1993). Indeed, research findings have shown that emotion-focused coping, including the unconscious process of denial and avoidance behavior, is not necessarily maladaptive or ineffective in certain traumatic encounters. Conversely, even when the situation at large is uncontrollable and a time of uncertainty and helplessness prevails, children need not restrict themselves solely to emotion-focused coping and can become involved in helpful prosocial activities in the aftermath of a disaster. (See Chapter 12 for other illustrations of active coping activities.)

Three major coping perspectives can be described in terms of timing and certainty: proactive, anticipatory, and reactive. *Proactive coping* constitutes the efforts undertaken in advance of a potentially stressful event to prevent it or to modify it before it develops (Aspinwall & Taylor, 1997). During the pre-impact preparatory phase, individuals and organizations proactively prepare to manage various unknown risks in a distant future by building up a broad range of coping behaviors and general stress resistance resources. Personal generic resistance resources comprise stress inoculation, learned optimism, the development of other life skills, and so on, whereas organizational generic resistance resources include long-term planning and resource accumulation.

Anticipatory coping refers to a person's premeditative efforts to manage (i.e., reduce, minimize, master, or tolerate) an impending stressful transaction (Lazarus & Folkman, 1984). During the second disaster phase (anticipatory warning phase), individuals instigate anticipatory coping aimed mainly at managing relatively known or expected risks, solving actual problems, reframing situations, and investing resources to counteract (i.e., prevent or minimize) the defined stressor or its risks. *Reactive coping* involves efforts to deal with a stressful encounter that is ongoing or has already happened. Individuals and organizations cope reactively during three phases of disaster: the impact phase, immediate postdisaster phase, and recovery phase. Giving forethought to coping in terms of timing and certainty sets the stage for integrative school-based programs at both the individual and organizational levels. Whereas the school organization must set aside time and resources for proactive and anticipatory organizational measures, many individual pupil-focused coping measures can be integrated into the regular curricula.

Practically speaking, essential useful characteristics of the recovery environment comprise allowing and supporting children to engage in emotion-focused activities and, concomitantly, helping them recognize and act upon elements of the environment that are responsive to their actions (Vernberg, 1999). It is our view that children should first be encouraged to use their preferred personal modes of responding to disaster and trauma. Modeling of useful coping strategies by significant adults (parents and teachers) may help children vicariously expand their repertoire. When necessary, students should be directly helped to enlarge and expand on their coping modes by trying to adopt or create new alternative strategies. Such interventions include guidance in accepting what is beyond one's control, while also coping creatively with situation-specific demands.

HABITUATING TO ADVERSITY

Habituation may provide one explanation for findings showing that children exhibit a high level of adaptation to war and warlike situations

(Klingman et al., 1993). Habituation refers to a decline in the tendency to respond to stimuli that have become familiar due to repeated exposure. The classic example consists of children's wide-range adaptation to air raids during the World War II blitz on London (Janis, 1951); the residents of London were reported also to demonstrate an adaptation of their sleep patterns to the circumstances (Pai, 1969). Israeli society can serve as another example. This society suffers from continuous exposure to threats to its security and even existence, unresolved economic strain, and the need to deal with the complex problems associated with mass immigration (Horowitz & Lissak, 1989). Nevertheless, many studies on Israeli children have shown less negative outcomes during adversity than may have been predicted, suggesting that habituation forces may be at work. For instance, studies conducted in a sleep laboratory in Israel during the 1991 Gulf War revealed that children who were awakened by the alarm siren indicating a missile attack were able to resume sleep without any evidence of persistent insomnia (Lavie, 2001). Similarly, schoolchildren's reports concerning their experience in the sealed room during the 1991 Gulf War indicated that, despite a shared feeling of high tension, the basic emotional stance was a positive form of detached optimism (Weisenberg, Schwarzwald, Waysman, Solomon, & Klingman, 1993). Likewise, Ziv and Israeli (1973) found that the anxiety level of children living on communal kibbutz settlements that suffered frequent enemy shelling did not significantly surpass that of children living on kibbutzim that were never under fire. The researchers suggested that the recurring stressor over time seemed to facilitate the development of adaptive defenses. However, another possible explanation could be the kibbutz's cohesive peer group and attentive caregivers, providing high levels of closeness, affiliation, and mutual support that may have facilitated children's adjustment.

Findings concerning ASD symptomatology in adolescents support the notion of habituation. During the second week of a 17-day massive rocket attack on an Israeli city (Klingman, 2001a), only 6% of the adolescents (grades 7 to 11) met all three ASD criteria. These adolescents reported a dominant sense of coping and adjustment, despite the circumstances. Hsu, Chong, Yang, and Yen (2002) found a relatively low rate of full PTSD among adolescents in Taiwan following an earthquake. They explained their finding in terms of the prolonged national security situation facing their country (similarly to Israel). They suggested that people in countries under long-term outside threat to their national security may develop coping and adaptation mechanisms to handle forthcoming traumatic events with marked resilience.

To explain habituation, Rachman (1990) suggested that people commonly initially *over-predict* the extent of anxiety they will experience in a novel adverse situation. However, with repeated disconfirmation of their over-prediction, their evaluations become more realistic, so that the situation becomes more predictable and more controllable. An alternative explanation, the *immunization model* (Breznitz, 1983), uses the analogy of the action of antibodies in the biological system. People develop, as it were, psychological antibodies and therefore emerge from their ordeal emotionally stronger. The question remains, though, as to the price imposed in the long run by habituation.

RESILIENCY BUILDING

The term *resiliency* generally refers to a class of phenomena characterized by patterns of positive adaptation in the context of significant unusual adversity or risk (Masten & Reed, 2002). Resiliency includes attitudes, coping behaviors, and personal strengths that are observed in people who "bounce back" from a stressful aversive situation and adjust well (Caspi, Bolger, & Eckenrode, 1987). The resiliency of a school may be addressed in terms of a sense of readiness, faith, commitment, ideology, and communality.

Antonovsky (1990) isolated a common dominator for resilience – the *sense of coherence* – to explain some persons' ability to cope well even in the face of horrific experiences, such as Nazi concentration camps, powerful discrimination, or abject poverty. The sense of coherence construct consists of comprehensibility (one's internal and external environments are predictable, structured, and explicit), manageability (resources are available and adequate), and meaningfulness (demands are worthy of investment and engagement). Although a sense of coherence is basically a personality disposition shaped by life experience until it stabilizes, cognitive-behavioral interventional mechanisms may enhance an efficacious coping style associated with a strong sense of coherence (Amirkhan & Greaves, 2003).

Three interrelated domains influence the manifestation of resilience: the child, family, and wider social environment. Resilience-promoting inner characteristics of the child may include easy inborn temperament, proficient social skills, or an ability to implement effective coping strategies. Such inner resources result in a higher level of self-esteem, a more realistic sense of personal control, and a feeling of optimism and hope. The family advances resilience when the home contains attributes like warmth, affection, emotional support, and clear-cut and reasonable rules. Finally, certain qualities of the larger social environment may foster resilience, such as the presence of other, charismatic adults who believe in and foster a strong, positive relationship with the child or the opportunity to develop a competency such as playing a musical instrument, volunteering with the elderly, babysitting, taking care of pets, or gardening (Merlone & Green, 2001).

BENEFIT-FINDING AND TRAUMA-INDUCED GROWTH

Some children go beyond mere resilience and actually rise above adversity to become stronger human beings. These youngsters "constructively confront" the traumatic experience (Moos, 2002) and emerge boasting greater self-confidence, new coping skills, maturation, closer ties with family and friends, and a noted change in their appreciation of life (Taylor & Wang, 2000). This phenomenon of *trauma-induced growth* – positive outcomes that can emerge from a person's struggle with a traumatic event (Calhoun & Tedeschi, 1999) – coincides with the positive psychology approach.

Individuals' discovery of benefits arising from their negative experiences has shown adaptive value (Tennen & Affleck, 2002). The notion that critical life problems offer possibilities for positive change is not new but has only recently been systematically investigated. Calhoun and Tedeschi (1999) outlined three major domains for posttraumatic growth: changes in relationships (increased compassion, more emotional sharing, greater attribution of importance); changes in the sense of self (self-perception as strong and capable of handling subsequent traumas); and changes in life philosophy (greater appreciation for everyday things, shifts in priorities, a new purpose in life). After the 9/11 attacks, for example, Americans reported becoming kinder, more grateful, and more spiritual. Data from an online questionnaire developed by Peterson and Seligman (2003) revealed a significant increase in six virtues they surveyed: love, gratitude, hope, kindness, spirituality, and teamwork. Although the long-term durability of this phenomenon needs to be examined further, it may remain high as long as the threat is in effect. In another study following the 9/11 attacks, college students reported a relatively low level of symptoms associated with ASD and an increase in trauma-induced growth or resiliency indicators. Most of the respondents reported new priorities in their lives, new respect for people in their communities, and a stronger appreciation for each day. They discovered that they were stronger than they had thought and learned that they could count on others in times of trouble (Sattler, 2003).

With regard to relationships, Breznitz (1983) highlighted the social benefit of a traumatic event as a "great integrator." Indeed, in our experience during times of school crisis or duress, we have also observed increasing social cohesion among students and among the teaching staff, a breakdown of traditional social barriers, and people closing ranks and supporting each other more than usual. Thus, what are bad times in one sense are often the best of times in another sense. At times of community crisis, individuals also may strongly identify with and relate to larger social units such as the extended family, peers, city, and even the entire nation or world. As a case in point, note the national unity that emerged after the 9/11 terrorist attacks in the USA or the staunch sense of identification experienced then by citizens in the United Kingdom and in many other western societies.

Facilitation of trauma-induced growth can be accomplished within the general framework of trauma-related interventions by encouraging the re-creation or construction of narrative, supporting a hopeful stance toward the future, and suggesting how to search for and find meaning and pur-pose. To creatively explore diverse means that allow for the gradual enhancement of trauma-induced growth, teachers and parents can encour-age cognitive processing of the trauma while highlighting that some poss-ible unnoticed positive benefits can occur out of experiences of vulnerability or weakness. For background materials, the teacher may util-ize relevant academic curricula and newspaper clippings about positive personal stories. By encouraging student interaction and peer support in the group, the teacher may further promote trauma-induced growth via social and interpersonal channels. (See teacher-mediated classroom crisis interventions in Chapter 11, positive expressive activities in Chapter 12, and also Tedeschi & Calhoun, 1995.)

An important aspect of benefit-finding and trauma-induced growth con-cerns their timing. Positive outcomes may emerge only after a process of emotional assimilation that follows an initial stage of emotional disorgani-zation, and positive outcomes may be accessed more readily when the stressors are perceived as more manageable (Stewart, Sokol, Healy, & Chester, 1986). These positive developments tend to emerge later in the recovery process; thus, efforts to encourage them immediately, or too early, after the event may be viewed as inept and insensitive by victims.

Part **II**

Multisystemic Interventions in Schools

Conceptual Basis for School-Wide Preventative Intervention

T he conceptual basis for our intervention guidelines and suggestions relates both to generic principles related to common needs around coping with trauma, as well as to essential considerations of group characteristics according to age, culture, and special needs. These will be presented in the following two chapters.

Chapter 9

The Generic Intervention Approach and Principles

S chool-based response to a disaster is *generic* in nature. The generic approach focuses on the characteristic course of the particular crisis, rather than on the unique response and the unique needs of each individual in crisis. The generic approach purports that an individual-focused approach – emphasizing individuals' unique, diverse intrapsychic and interpersonal processes and needs – can always be initiated later on if necessary, based on a careful screening and referral process. Yet, the generic approach first recognizes certain common response patterns to mass disaster, that is, normal reactions to abnormal circumstances. According to this approach, an intervention should therefore first be directed toward an adaptive resolution of the crisis. This is not to say that psychological problems associated with maladaptive coping will not evolve, but rather that the intervention must first ensure that people's adaptive coping is activated. Moreover, individual-focused intervention in the early phase of the disaster may be premature or undesirable because it can amplify a problem that may disappear spontaneously or through generic intervention, and thus lead to unnecessary psychological labeling and stigma. Thus, large-scale school-based intervention measures employed immediately after a disaster should be designed to be effective for all members of a given group, rather than to focus on the unique attributes of each individual (Aguilera & Messic, 1978). The individual-focused approach is used subsequently if individuals fail to respond to generic measures, and thus complements the generic intervention.

Our rather extensive experience with large-scale disasters has shown us that generic intervention principles closely resembling those employed for soldiers suffering from combat stress reactions (e.g., Artiss, 1963) provide great benefit when applied in schools and other community settings. These optimal generic intervention principles comprise immediacy, proximity, psychological sense of community, expectancy, simplicity, purposeful action, and the unifying principle of continuity.

The generic principle of *immediacy* accentuates the importance of ensuring that preventive measures are taken as soon as possible after impact, preventing hiatuses that would deepen the sense of disruption. Such measures include meeting immediate practical needs like physical shelter; food and drink, medical attention as well as psychoeducational needs, like a sense of safety and an opportunity to ventilate feelings and talk. The hours and days after a traumatic event (i.e., the impact and immediate postdisaster phases) should be viewed as the key period for generic intervention. If stress responses go unattended for a longer duration, adjustment difficulties will likely become more ingrained.

The generic principle of *proximity* implies the preference to intervene at the natural setting, or as close as possible to it, so as to protect people's existing personal networks within which they usually function. Studies of British children who experienced constant bombings and witnessed destruction, injury, or death during World War II (Freud & Burlingham, 1943; Janis, 1951) indicated little adverse effects, provided that children remained in the familiar setting with their regular caretakers and continued their familiar routines. Thus, this principle strongly advocates remaining in, or quickly returning to, the community and the school, whenever possible, rather than being separated (e.g., "sent away for a while") or avoiding the school by remaining at home. School-based postdisaster intervention thus intervenes in the natural setting and meets the proximity principle.

The generic principle of *sense of community* refers to involving all those similarly affected in joint interventions, usually conducted in a classroom or peer group setting. This principle espouses mobilizing the resources in the students' familiar school and community environments to serve as effective support systems, enhancing feelings of belongingness, and fostering a sense of relative stability. Such resources include peers, teachers, school counselors, family, youth leaders, and clergy.

The generic principle of *expectancy* involves establishing confidence in one's ability to recover. The school staff should clearly and systematically communicate and convey to the students and their families that they are expected (a) to recover, notwithstanding difficulties and problems, and (b) to gradually resume prior, pre-crisis duties, activities, and functioning.

The generic principle of *simplicity* implies that intervention methods should not be sophisticated and complicated but rather as simple as possible, with clear goals aimed at normalization of stress reactions. Such features include provision of rest, relaxation, information, opportunities for ventilation, attentive and sensitive listening, caring, and companionship. In essence, every person (i.e., not only a mental health professional) and every simple everyday activity can become "therapeutic" if utilized to help the organization and the individual advance toward recovery.

The principle of *purposeful action* implies that being active can serve as a powerful counter-response to helplessness. Based on laboratory studies, Ledoux and Gorman (2001) asserted that enhancement of *active coping* helps whenever one entertains dysphoric thoughts or avoids necessary and meaningful activities that may induce feelings of helplessness. Action enhances a sense of strength and induces expectancy for change and recovery. Thus, children should have opportunities (and in certain cases also be encouraged) to become involved in simple, purposeful activities. Action is more rewarding when focused on a cause and when not too difficult. Engaging in an overly challenging or complex task in a fearful context may lead to a state of immobility. Devotion to a cause, however minimal, creates a feeling of togetherness, joint commitment, and positive expectancy.

THE UNIFYING CONTINUITY PRINCIPLE

The *continuity principle* may be considered the unifying generic guiding principle. It stipulates that large-scale disaster situations cause extreme disruption in both everyday personal and community life and may shatter basic schemata such as beliefs in one's invulnerability and faith in the predictability, manageability, and meaningfulness of the world (Alon & Levine Bar-Yoseph, 1994; Klingman, 2001b; Omer & Alon, 1994). Indeed, schoolchildren may experience interruptions in school activities and functions, changes in family routines and roles, and suspension or even loss of habitual social responsibilities and activities. This principle further asserts that, to counteract these acute disruptions, disaster and trauma management should aim at preserving and restoring functional, historical, and interpersonal continuities at the individual, familial, organizational, and community levels, at all stages of the problem cycle, as follows:

School Organizational Continuity

A school crisis intervention guided by the continuity principle will thus consider continuity of the school organization to be a most important prevention factor of highest priority. School organizational continuity entails the restoration of the connection between students and their natural school environment and the restoration of the school as a functioning organization. According to the continuity principle, the school's crisis team, with the help of expert mental health professionals, must first reach out to both administrative staff and teachers to help them resume their roles and reinstate disrupted familiar school routines. The team serves as facilitator of situation-relevant reorganization by helping the school staff and administration to realize their strengths, by probing and processing immediate solutions to problems, and also by devising situation-tailored structured activities that rebuild the students' sense of stability, order, and continuity.

Personal Continuity

The preservation or restoration of one's sense of self-identity as well as one's identity in relation to the family, school, and community can be achieved through age-appropriate cognitive and emotional working-through. Individuals must gradually process and integrate the event into their world perceptions to ascertain that life before the event, the event itself, its meaning, their responses to it, and life after it all become part of a meaningful continuum. Interventions promoting personal continuity help uncover causal explanations for the event, reconstruct the meaning of the individual's life around the setbacks involved, and preserve or restore personal identity through rituals and expressive means.

Functional Continuity

A close complement to personal continuity, functional continuity comprises the ability to continue to fulfill individual, familial, academic, or organizational roles and activities despite the disruption. In the school setting, this refers to the gradual restoration of pre-crisis roles and duties (e.g., as a school principal, a teacher, and a pupil) and to gaining a sense of mastery by exerting behavioral control over some, however small, aspects of the threat-related issues and of everyday school life. Functional continuity involves encouraging children to take prosocial action and to resume their pre-crisis (school-related, social, familial) roles and activities whenever possible. It begins with taking even symbolic, very simple steps towards the resumption of their previous functioning, then gradually broadening the scope and complexity of assignments and functional demands.

Interpersonal Continuity

Survivors of disaster must continue their ability to maintain and use interpersonal significant ties and, when needed, to use them for obtaining and offering support. Interpersonal continuity concerns reestablishing pre-crisis social bonds, and thus enhancing a sense of communality and gaining a feeling of group solidarity as an antidote to possible forthcoming difficulties. Reinvesting in interpersonal relationships with peers and teachers provides social support, which has been found to be beneficial to recovery. Such reinvestment also plays an important role in counteracting the possible loss of faith in human beings, especially following deliberate, violent human disasters. When a school is temporarily closed and face-to-face contacts are not possible, the contacts between pupils and school staff and peers can be reestablished by telephone and e-mail. The return to school as soon as possible enables reunions with peers and teachers, thus reestablishing the predisaster level of daily social interactions. School and classroom group work around emotional reactions to the disaster and some disaster-related topics are helpful in drawing children and staff closer together again.

Continuity of Care

This aspect, derived from a mental health care frame of reference, can be added to the continuity principle. Continuity of care ideally relates to the provision of a range of accessible multimodal preventive interventions and the need for mental health professionals to systematically, routinely, and periodically assess reactions and symptoms in all children. Importantly, this aspect of continuity identifies children who continue to exhibit trauma-related symptoms or do not spontaneously report their symptoms, as well as those who develop delayed symptoms. Continuity of care is optimally implemented in the school setting where all children can be involved, both directly and indirectly, in preventive activities, and also can be systematically observed and assessed at different points in time. This most demanding responsibility can be more realistically accomplished when it is shared both by the teaching staff and mental health faculty, provided they have been properly trained in identifying posttraumatic reactions.

Chapter 10

Developmental, Functional, and Cultural Considerations

Any school-based intervention must incorporate special considerations relating to developmental variables, children's special needs, and multicultural factors.

DEVELOPMENTAL CONSIDERATIONS

Ample reason exists to believe that children's developmental level renders multiple and profound effects on the ways in which disasters are experienced as well as on possible outcomes elicited by disasters (La Greca et al., 2002). A central concern should be the subjective meaning of the traumatic event for each child, within that child's level of conceptual understanding. The students' ability to interpret more accurately the degree of threat posed by the objective events emerges gradually with age. Variables such as the child's knowledge base and language development influence how the adverse event is encoded, appraised, and represented in memory.

Preschool and Elementary School Students

A number of variables typify younger children in comparison to their older counterparts. Younger children encode the traumatic event with less detail and experience more gaps and distortions in memory than do older children. Consequently, the younger child's account is vulnerable to omissions and other errors. Their lower capability of relating to cause-and-effect also may lead to a failure in accurately appraising the experience. Language development at the time of encoding also significantly influences the extent to which an experience can be verbalized. Affect regulation, in terms of the threshold for arousal and tolerance for arousal, also correlates with age (van der Kolk, 1997). In addition, inhibition of the startle reflex continues to develop through middle childhood, and the ability to attend to multiple dimensions of experience (e.g., internal cues and environmental symbols) improves only with age. Thus, younger children can be very frightened by events that produce only mild fear in adolescents and adults, attend more selectively or idiosyncratically to signals of threat, and be strongly influenced by reactions of adults, especially attachment figures (La Greca et al., 2002).

Only around middle childhood do youngsters master the ability to adopt a range of cognitive strategies likely to influence their covert and overt responses and select strategies for coping with particular problems including the regulation of emotions. Before middle childhood, students tend not to initiate talk about past events because of memory factors and lack of experience with the narrative form to guide their retrieval and reporting, which may deprive them of a means for re-appraising the experience and correcting misconceptions. They may also give "magical" explanations to fill in the gaps in understanding. They may express concerns (openly or subtly) about the safety of self and significant others and may be preoccupied with danger. Immaturity in social cognition, memory, and language and conversation may protect the younger students from negative symptoms; however, these children are susceptible to cues from the adults around them and thus influenced by their reactions. Hence, high anxiety and helplessness levels in adults may result in diminished means of coping with the adverse experience.

Preschool students especially need substantial assistance in identifying their "feeling vocabulary," so that they can verbalize their distress. For them, hands-on activities are most helpful to express feelings nonverbally. Most interventions at this stage involve playing as well as other symbolic activities; play enables them to re-enact the traumatic event, divide the overwhelming and painful experiences into small quantities, experience ventilation of feelings, work feelings through, symbolize and modify consequences, and gradually assimilate the experience into their existing schemas (Bevin, 1991), allowing them to follow their own pace.

By the age of 8 or 9, children's fears show an increasing cognitive awareness of real dangers to self and significant others. Children at this age may be extremely concerned about the safety and security of their caretakers and demonstrate an acute preoccupation with the loss of personal possessions or pets. The children's cognitive development enables them to link two events and begin to better understand the concept of death; thus, elementary school children can more fully comprehend the scope and intensity of an event. However, children at this age may also continue to use magical thinking when feeling a loss of control.

Adults play important roles in helping young students manage their emotions, providing them with information and simplified narratives to interpret experiences for them, and selecting appropriate situations and showing them coping options. However, some teachers refrain from dealing with events in class as a means of protecting young children from further upset, or when teachers underestimate or do not realize the full extent of the students' distress, or because of the teachers' own high level of distress. This should receive the attention of the mental health consultant.

Preadolescent and Adolescent Students

At preadolescence, peer awareness and peer relationships occupy students; disruption of school life may disrupt their peer relationships. At this developmental stage, students' cognitive maturity enables them to understand and conceptualize more abstract and existential issues such as accountability, survivor guilt, alternative actions, their own limitations, loss of life, and loss of significant others (Stallard, 2000). Adolescents exhibit more awareness of and concern with their bodies, physical intactness, and the threat of disfigurement.

Inasmuch as adolescents strive to appear independent, strong, and competent to the world around them, they may refrain from discussing overwhelming emotions with adults to avoid showing dependency and weakness. They may be especially reluctant to seek out counseling. In certain cases, they may challenge, resist, and disagree with adults to the point of aggressive behavior.

Adolescents tend to respond even more to the world beyond their families; thus ideology, patriotism, and ideological commitment become more compelling. As a result, teenagers may be intolerant and suspicious of peers from a different racial, ethnic, or religious background, or due to peers' non-conforming behavior. They may also adopt a revenge-oriented ideology as a simplistic mechanism for coping. Thus, teachers (especially in social studies) must ensure that the topic of tolerance is explored. This was dramatically noted following the 9/11 attack; as fear over the event transformed to anger, the intensification of hatred toward Muslims appeared among students. Teachers then focused on Muslim teachings to counter misperceptions and misconceptions about Islamic scriptures and beliefs (i.e., that there is no jurisprudence for indiscriminate killings or assassinations of local or foreign citizens by either Sunni or Shiite Muslims).

Adolescents' developmental tasks include planning for the future, creating intimate relationships, relating to the world, and mastering conflicting moral questions and complex cause-effect circumstances. Adolescents may worry about their future and the fate of the world or may become fearful of leaving home, viewing the world as unsafe. In contrast, they might exhibit feelings of omnipotence, altruism, and a strong need to abolish injustice. Teenagers' tendency for risk-taking behaviors may lead to irresponsible actions and even dangerous conduct. They may dare to approach dangerous areas and think it courageous to handle dangerous objects left in the aftermath of a disaster.

Onset of PTSD symptomatology in this phase may have particularly negative implications for the acquisition and mastery of adolescent life skills (e.g., separation, emancipation, self-identity, and vocational interest). In addition, PTSD-related symptoms of avoidance and numbing may interfere with social relationships and thus impair the ability to forge meaningful interpersonal ties.

The developmental considerations mentioned refer to the common patterns of growth. However, appreciation of individual differences is most important. Cognitive capacity and growth is not unitary. Children have multiple and varied "intelligences;" genetic influences exist for diversity as well as for similarity; and individual children achieve the ability to perform various tasks at very different rates according to their genetic make-up.

CHILDREN WITH SPECIAL NEEDS

The situation-specific condition of children with special needs should draw our attention in intervention planning. Very little research or writing is available about the reactions of children with special needs to large-scale disasters. The needs of students with learning disabilities may not differ from those of their non-disabled peers, but some possible specific deficits should be addressed. For example, children with attention deficit disorder (ADD) or attention deficit hyperactivity disorder (ADHD) may misread social cues and miss messages concerning their safety. They may have difficulty following the sequence of events as repeated again and again on television, or not understand the complexities of the situation. Some children with learning disabilities may interpret language very literally; others who have difficulty with temporal and spatial concepts may be confused by what they hear and see around them and in the media.

Following the 9/11 attacks, the U.S. National Association of School Psychologists (NASP) produced a handout for caregivers that touched upon the issue of special needs (National Association of School Psychologists, 2003). Their basic assumption was that school educators who are most familiar with the child who has special needs can best know and best predict that child's reactions and behaviors based on prior observation of the child in different stressful situations. NASP also asserted the appropriateness of many available crisis response resources for use with students who have disabilities, provided that individual consideration is given to the child's physical developmental and emotional capabilities. Some students may need to be more protected or isolated to minimize distraction and sources of agitation during the height of a traumatic event.

MULTICULTURAL CONSIDERATIONS

Schools in postmodern society serve an increasingly culturally diverse student and family population. Cultural factors play an important role in individuals' or groups' expression of stress reactions, vulnerability to developing PTSD, and treatment responsiveness. Trauma responses do share some universal features; however, cultural groups may handle stressors differently. For example, social sharing of emotion is a cross-cultural phenomenon, but the sharing modalities show cultural differences. Marked differences exist regarding what is considered useful or acceptable in responding to disaster. Variables such as sense of community, needs and preferences for certain types of help, motivation, sense of privacy, honor and pride regarding the involvement of psychological help, political systems, leadership patterns, and political leaders' involvement are but a few of the variables affected by cultural differences. Emotional expression, considered to enhance recovery in one culture, may represent self-indulgence, weakness, disrespect, and brashness in another. Encouragement for emotional self-expression may not yield the expected response in children of a culture that does not legitimize it. In other cultures, public shouting, trembling, and seizure-like episodes, observed especially at funerals, comprise culture-bound syndromes that serve to mobilize the support of the social network.

Cross-cultural aspects of grief illuminate on the role of the family and grief rituals across cultures. Although feelings of grief accompany losses everywhere and are considered a "core grieving process" that occurs across cultures (Rosenblat, 1993), considerable evidence indicates that cultural (and religious) beliefs influence the meaning of death. Funerary practices that govern the expression of emotions can radically alter peoples' emotional reaction to bereavement. For example, individuals from non-Western societies often express their emotional difficulties through somatization (Al-Krenawi & Graham, 2000; Dwairy, 1998). Cultural beliefs can restore the bereaved to a positive sense of self by such means as recreating a relationship with the deceased as a spirit-being; religious beliefs can make pain less threatening by giving suffering meaning within a larger moral order (Al-Krenawi, Graham, & Sehwail, 2002). However, emotional needs may conflict with role expectations; for example, although grief constitutes a natural way for discharge of emotions following the death of a loved one, widows of Palestinian martyrs are expected (and often pressured) to rejoice at their husband's death (Sande, 1998).

Nonverbal as well as verbal communication variations are also noted. Gestures and physical contact typical to a particular culture can be misleading if not recognized. In some cultures, personal questions are considered intrusive or eye contact during communication is not acceptable. Physical contact (e.g., touching, embracing) between helper and a child or adolescent is viewed in some cultures as appropriate following a traumatic event, as it assists (especially children) in crisis to feel comforted and less alone; however, it may be inappropriate or even unacceptable in other cultures (Sandoval & Lewis, 2002). In addition, the nuances of specific words, phrases, slogans, or proverbs may be incorrectly interpreted. Crisis responders should attempt to understand their own cultural identities as well as their cultural biases when they reach out to help others.

A noted culturally determined obstacle in trauma intervention is the very strong resistance to mental health professionals and to the entire concept of mental health intervention. Attempts to help may be misunderstood as meddling, interference, or even political attempts to influence or control (Dohrty, 1999). Firmly rooted in some cultures are beliefs that one ought to have no personal problems, or that one must present a strong face to the outside world, or that the mere fact of seeing a mental health professional might cause one to be labeled "ill." Such a culture may reject or stigmatize traumatized people, which may cause them additional injury.

Cultures also offer strengths in coping with trauma. The routines, traditions, and rituals imbedded in a particular culture may aid traumatized people who belong to that culture by defining culture-dependent pathways to recovery. For example, each culture has its own relevant way for explaining death and searching for the meaning of suffering and pain. Culture-bound rituals and religious rites act as a healthy expression of a wide range of trauma-related contents, as they have a cathartic effect. They serve to enable emotional release and expression through attachment and connection to significant others as well. Rituals and rites also enhance a structured, gradual move towards adaptation and trauma-induced growth. In some cultural contexts, religious leaders, ritual specialists, or traditional healers play a pivotal role in constructing a shared sense of reality and meaning.

In contrast to the Western mental health approaches' focus on the individual, non-Western collectivist cultures focus on the family and the traditional group. A more traditional "we – self" intervention may prove more relevant, accessible, and effective than the "I – self" one. Multilingual materials and culturally relevant messages that are endorsed and delivered by persons from the specific culture who have local respect and authority may help ensure that preventive intervention measures are successfully disseminated and followed. Interventions with victims may need the involvement of a "culture-broker" from the affected cultural group. A mental health professional culture-broker is preferable to laymen "translators" who may refrain from translating messages because of perceived cultural insult to one or another of the parties involved in the interchange (Stamm & Friedman, 2000).

In sum, recovery can be facilitated through knowledge and sensitivity to the particular characteristics of culturally different students and their parents or guardians, when providing trauma intervention.

Interventions for Students, Staff, and Families

This section focuses on the organizational procedures and measures, psychoeducational techniques, and instructional activities employed by various school personnel to counter the hazards of trauma. Basic guidelines and ideas for activities and interventions are offered according to a comprehensive model, which is responsive to the changing demands at the various stages of the traumatic event, and to the accompanying coping and processing needs.

Chapter 11

School-Based 7-Level Preventive Intervention Model

Prevention basically entails undertaking action to (a) forestall development of a problem in the first place, (b) identify a problem sufficiently early in its developmental course, (c) reduce unnecessary suffering related to the problem, and (d) activate a myriad of interventions to promote (internal as well as external) resistance resources for at-risk populations. In the school context, prevention must be directed at four target groups: students, educational staff, administrative/support staff, and parents. The school-based preventive crisis response must first and foremost invest efforts in restoring equilibrium. To accomplish this, the school must, first, offer its population new alternatives for dealing both with the troubling situation and with the stresses it creates and, second, adapt school practices so as to ensure appropriate reorganization that provides situation-specific recovery measures.

Caplan (1964) coined the definitive three-tiered general classification of preventive psychiatry into primary prevention, secondary prevention, and tertiary prevention. Utilizing Caplan's classification, the first author of this book (Klingman) constructed a typological multi-level preventive intervention model to meet the specific needs of school reorganization around disaster response (Klingman, 1988, 1993, 1996, 2001a). This typological model consists of seven preventive intervention levels constituting a comprehensive and coordinated disaster response plan, comprising:

- Crisis preparedness
- Anticipatory guidance
- Postdisaster immediate organizational response
- Primary preventive intervention
- Early secondary preventive intervention
- Indicated secondary preventive intervention

- Tertiary preventive intervention

This model refers to levels rather than stages because the latter imply a progression or chronological development, whereas these seven levels can partially overlap or concur in time. Using this 7-level model, this chapter will present our recommended practical guidelines for systematic school-activated preventive interventions and will particularly elaborate on issues related to their implementation in the pre- and early postdisaster periods.

CRISIS PREPAREDNESS LEVEL

The preparatory level aims at strengthening the school as a system as well as the individuals within it to better cope with disaster if and when it occurs. This level refers mainly to measures and interventions that will eventually foster the organizational, behavioral, and mental schemata needed for efficient transition between routine (non-disaster) and emergency functioning (e.g., disaster warning, disaster impact), if and when disaster strikes.

At the school crisis preparatory level, as an integral part of their everyday operation, schools should develop school-wide organizational and curricular approaches that include resiliency building as well as prepare specific crisis responses focusing on what to do when a crisis emerges. As we stressed earlier, preventative investment in both resiliency building and a disaster response plan during quiet times can meaningfully contribute to school functioning and student adjustment in the impact and post-impact periods of an actual, potentially traumatic event.

Resiliency Building

Conceptually, *resiliency building* can be associated with the universal preventive interventions classified by the Committee on Prevention of Mental Disorders of the Institute of Medicine (Mrazek & Haggerty, 1994), which benefit a wide population that has not been identified on the basis of individual risk. Several researchers have asserted the value of preparatory programs for general coping with stress (e.g., Janis, 1951; Meichenbaum & Cameron, 1983). School-based resiliency building should aim to strengthen all three of the following interrelated domains: the inner resources of the child, the family, and the larger social environment (e.g., school and community). Interventions targeting the individual's inner resources would include training in problem-solving skills, social skills, and coping strategies for dealing with situational as well as developmental life stressors. In the larger social domain, a caring, nurturing school staff can provide students with experiences that enhance self-esteem and strategies reinforcing hope and resilience (Brooks, 2002).

Schools should thus invest daily in developing effective coping skills of students and staff and in improving the classroom and school climate, via programs such as peer counseling, violence prevention, peer mediation, conflict resolution, and aggression replacement training. Specific, school-based structured programs may (with some modifications) follow programs like the Stress Inoculation Program (Meichenbaum & Cameron, 1983), the Penn Resiliency/Optimism Program (Gillham, Reivich, & Shatte, 2001; Seligman, Reivich, Jaycox, & Gillham, 1995), or more problem-specific programs such as the prevention of self-destructive behaviors (e.g., Klingman & Hochdorf, 1993). Resiliency building by a focus on optimal well-being can contribute indirectly to a better ability to overcome stress, frustration, and problems.

Disaster Preparedness Planning

The crisis management aspect of preparedness targets school staff and concerns the how and what to do in each specific school when crisis emerges. School disaster preparedness requires the initiation and development of a comprehensive crisis response plan built upon both in-school and off-campus resources. The plan's development entails organizational, emotional/social, and functional components. *Organizational preparedness* involves forming a planning committee; designing clear, adaptable, functional, and flexible physical response options as well as administrative procedures to meet the school's needs during disaster and its aftermath; organizing a school crisis response team; developing liaison and coordination with significant community support agencies; and establishing a written user-friendly crisis management guide or manual. *Emotional/social preparedness* involves in-service preparation that focuses on processing of feelings and thoughts related to past and future disaster and trauma in a supportive group, as well as on identifying both personal and interpersonal resources for crisis intervention. *Functional preparedness* refers to activities aimed at training and examining the efficacy of the crisis response plan, via simulation.

Although advocated more than two decades ago (e.g., Klingman, 1978), the notion of a school-based crisis intervention plan remained in its infancy a decade ago. However, recently, the public has come to expect school crisis readiness, and policy makers have been increasingly mandating today's schools to better prepare for possible disasters (Brock & Poland, 2002). Currently, a variety of resources about initiating and implementing a crisis response plan are available to schools as they embark on crisis preparedness (e.g., Brock & Poland, 2002; Brock, Sandoval, & Lewis, 2001; Lichtenstein, Schonfeld, Kline, & Speese-Lineham, 1995), and a variety of sample school plans can also be downloaded from the Internet.

Next, we will elaborate on five of the main tasks for crisis preparedness: developing a core school planning committee; preparing a school-based crisis response plan and manual; school disaster proofing; setting up the school crisis intervention team; and undertaking crisis education, simulations and drills.

The Core Crisis Response Planning Committee

The first major organizational and functional task in crisis response preparation entails the school's formation of a relatively small *core crisis response planning committee*. The committee's tasks encompass the initiation and development of a crisis response plan, a written crisis management guide/manual, and a larger school crisis response team (and its task-designated sub-teams). Steps suggested for the planning committee include determining goals, performing needs assessment, examining model programs, and designating a base of operations on the school campus (Purvis, Porter, Authement, & Boren, 1991).

Members of the core planning committee are recruited by the school administration and serve by role and interest. Committee members should have a diverse and complementary knowledge base as well as acquaintance with relevant school management and crisis intervention skills. At a minimum, the committee should consist of a leading administrator (e.g., principal or assistant principal), teaching staff representatives (e.g., homeroom teacher, special education teacher), mental health professional representatives (e.g., in-school counseling services coordinator, school psychologist), a representative of the maintenance staff, and a parent liaison (a knowledgeable parent representative such as chairperson of the school parent-teacher association – PTA). It is also advisable to have a representative of the businesses or residences neighboring the school.

The school mental health professional, regardless of his or her later role on the committee, can assume leadership and start the process rolling by presenting first to the school administration, and then to the school staff, the rationale and psychological knowledge base supporting the need to invest in disaster preparation. This is an educational intervention intended to obtain the support of the administration and to motivate the staff to become actively involved. When introducing the need for a school preparedness plan, the mental health professional should emphasize its suitability for any school crisis (e.g., a student's suicidal risk, or the death of a teacher). Although, at times of need, the school may activate off-campus support services and external trauma experts, building a school crisis team with on-campus members offers strong advantages. School staff members maintain an ongoing relationship with and knowledge about each other and the school's particular students, parents, community, and available resources. Logistically, the school staff can also most easily meet on a routine basis to review the crisis plan and examine issues unique to the school. In addition, school staff members can systematically monitor emerging and residual effects of a disaster throughout the long recovery period

(Newgass & Schonfeld, 2000). Moreover, in large-scale disasters, it is diffi-cult to rely on community or district services, as they must often simul-taneously respond to needs in many schools.

The core crisis response planning committee also comprises the nucleus of the school-based crisis response team. After completing the plan and the written manual, the core planning committee expands to become the school *crisis response team* (see below). However, the planning committee remains as such when adding new protocols and when reevaluating and possibly revising the older ones periodically.

Preparing a School-Based Crisis Response Plan and Manual

The *school-based crisis response plan* constitutes the major product of the core planning committee. Over a series of meetings and discussions, the committee develops a set of written practical guidelines, prepared in the form of a hands-on manual, to be followed in school drills and simulations, in staff education and training, and when disaster strikes. Obviously, this manual serves mainly as a blueprint for administrators regarding organi-zational response needs, and for teachers to help them respond to stu-dents' needs. However, the needs of the school staff (administrative, educational, and support staff), parents, and mental health personnel themselves should not be overlooked, in order to enable them to enlist their own strengths and available resources for handling the crisis.

Furthermore, the crisis response manual must address the roles and dif-ficulties of the non-teaching school support staff. The school secretary, librarian, custodian, lunch server, cleaners, and nurse may play a pivotal role in handling crisis situations, considering their informal relationships with students and the fact that they are often considered by many as "favo-rites" at school. Duties of office staff and other school support staff increase geometrically following trauma (Nader & Pynoos, 1993). This includes increased phone calls, secretarial services, paperwork, physical intrusion of officials, inflow of distressed parents, flooding by the press, and the like. Less noted but very important can be the role of school cus-todians. For example, amid chaos resulting from the September 11 WTC attack, custodians from the nearby Stuyvesant High School were reported to lend valuable helping hands in securing the school buildings, looking for needed emergency supplies, mopping up behind emergency workers, and setting up numerous tables and chairs in the school to serve as tem-porary headquarters for rescue forces. Thus, the crisis response plan can assign school support staff multiple tasks, but should also allocate them consultants' advice and psychological support (Lee, 2001).

The crisis response manual may also expand the school nurse's roles and responsibilities. The nurse's protocol can also include informing the rescue teams and educational staff of any prior health problems relevant to medical care or later recovery. The school nurse may play a pivotal role in triage and monitoring casualties during impact, and the mental health triage system after it, because schoolchildren often report increased somatic complaints after a seriously distressing event (Nader & Pynoos, 1993). The nurse may act in a number of roles: as a health professional, who can monitor students' recovery; a health resource person; an educator; and at times a counselor or confidante. Provisions can also be made in advance for the school nurse's office to serve as a *safe room* (Stevenson, 2002), to offset student absenteeism (see below).

The manual includes technical-procedural components, psychoeducational components, and strategic components.

The *technical-procedural components of the manual* should specify the pre-designated personnel (both school-based and school-linked) and the range of recommended organizational and educational procedures and activities to be followed in response to diverse disaster scenarios. These protocols include safety and security measures and means for disseminating information to staff, students, and parents. The manual also contains crucial information such as emergency telephone/e-mail/address lists of school personnel, students' families, and community emergency and support services. Schools also need to predesignate an appropriate space (and alternative locations) for a command post, in-school and alternative shelters, alternate absorption centers, locations for reuniting children and parents, and within-school support rooms to be staffed by counseling personnel for short-term individual or group support. All these should be clearly marked on a detailed and enlarged map of the school buildings and grounds, which should be included in the manual. In addition, the manual should include various procedures and escape routes for evacuation as well as protocols for securing access into and out of the building and grounds, for communicating with parents, and for controlling the flow of parents, volunteers, various agency representatives, and media personnel. Issues of interagency coordination and media management deserve prior attention when devising a crisis response plan.

The crisis response manual must address those well-intentioned agencies or individual professionals who may rush in to volunteer in the school, eliciting competing interests and conflicting professional attitudes. We recognize that this much-noted, persistent difficulty may constitute an unavoidable inherent problem in disaster management because of the rapidly changing conditions and often improvised interventions following a disaster. School personnel may feel that professional outsiders are intrusive in the school corridors and classrooms, usurping teachers' authority and causing disagreements (Toubiana, Milgram, Strich, & Edelstein, 1988). Thus, the postdisaster protocols should assign particular crisis team members the task of courteously monitoring "experts'" or other "outsiders'" school entry, or attempts to take on a direct active role, without prior coordination.

Interagency Collaboration

The *psychoeducational component of the manual* addresses the most common reactions to major stressful events in children, followed by a presentation of their age-related psychological needs. The mental health professional contributes the major input to this component of the manual. This section of the guidelines includes age-related typical and atypical reactions to traumatic experience, developmental and cultural considerations, and psychological first-aid principles and steps. In particular, procedures for funeral attendance, staff and student briefings, and curricular adjustments should be addressed. In addition, the mental health professional should review contents composed by other professionals and suggest relevant mental health aspects that should be integrated into these (e.g., trauma/disaster-related didactic materials and lesson plans). Short case examples of children's psychological responses, and outlines of school-and class-based interventions, may be very useful. This component of the manual will also include a list of community mental health services available to assist the school during times of crisis, a list of religious and cultural community liaison persons, as well as community services for trauma victims. The school's mental health professional and the core planning committee should pre-establish coordination procedures with these services. In addition, the manual should present in-school protocols and instruments for identifying and referring psychological trauma victims to the appropriate treatment.

The *strategic component of the manual* includes the basic assumptions underlying the intervention approach, the organizational procedures, generic response principles (see Chapter 9), intervention principles (e.g., strategies for facilitating class discussion), checklists, and sample forms (e.g., a letter to send home). The crisis management manual can also include vignettes for crisis team and sub-team training as well as samples for organization-oriented school-wide crisis simulation scenarios (also see: Lichtenstein et al., 1995, and later descriptions in this chapter of crisis education and simulations).

To best prepare for large-scale disaster, the planning committee should invite representatives of community or district agencies, which are in supervisory, collaborative, or supportive positions, to participate in committee discussions dealing with the procedures involving their coordinated actions. This coordination may involve the development, in advance, of protocols identifying procedures and key individuals, resources, and support groups in the community with whom collaboration has been pre-arranged. Such protocols must also include available local (formal and informal) resources for instances in which regional and district or community teams are not available, and the steps by which these resources can be mobilized when needed.

Pre-crisis interagency education, training, and coordination can reduce professionals' theoretical orientation differences (e.g., dynamic versus cognitive-behavioral treatment approaches), increase their familiarity with generic principles of crisis intervention, and resolve conflicts associated with actual or perceived overlapping jurisdictions. The consolidation of an agreed-upon conceptual and pragmatic "psychological language," and training in trauma-focused intervention methods are all of paramount importance for the execution of effective intervention in times of disaster (Nader & Pynoos, 1993).

In addition, every locality needs to reach agreement on a community-wide plan that encompasses its schools. In most instances, schools must follow district administration policy and detailed procedural guidelines for handling major disasters; therefore, any school-based planning must relate to the system-wide organizational (i.e., the regional and the district) disaster intervention plan.

Media Management

Disaster is a media event that brings victims, classmates, and educational and administrative staff into the headlines. Such exposure often involves public meddling into their private lives as well as school affairs. Media harassment of the school population can compound the trauma. It is thus vitally important that the school deliberately set out to organize press conferences, give well-informed information to media representatives that is consonant with the interests of the victims and the school, and thus also set the tone for future interaction with the media. The manual should pre-assign staff to carry out such tasks as ensuring that media personnel visit the school by invitation and appointment only. The crisis response plan should make provisions for the school staff responsible for media management to consult with the school's mental health professional about the contents and tone of communications with the media at that time. The school-designated media spokesperson can receive predisaster education on how to avoid pitfalls. Our experience suggests that whenever a school administration alienated the media, the latter emphasized sensational aspects of the event and directly and unselectively approached pupils, disturbing their privacy. A proactive approach by the school towards the media offers much potential benefit in providing a balanced presentation of the trauma effects, calming messages, and even some advice on positive coping.

School "Disaster Proofing"

One early organizational preparedness task that may be conducted by the school's core crisis response planning committee during their attempt to develop a crisis management plan comprises physical "disaster proofing." Schools should instigate an inspection of all their facilities to verify structural safety, identify safe zones for various emergencies (e.g., in the event of a hurricane or tornado), and establish alternative escape routes (e.g., for terrorist or sniper attack). This process may include gas-proofing certain spaces to ready them as sealed shelters in case of chemical attack. Such preparations may require securing the availability and approachability of basic medical first aid and other emergency supplies including food, battery-powered radio, telephone and television, an alternative drinking supply if water mains are disconnected, and activity materials and supplies (e.g., paper, pencils and crayons, puzzles, magazines) to be used in case of an extended stay in the shelter. The suitability of these emergency zones and supplies should be examined through drills and simulations.

The School Crisis Intervention Team

The core crisis response planning committee should recruit crisis intervention team members, based mostly on role and special expertise relevant to crisis intervention and crisis management. The crisis intervention or management team basically consists of a chairperson (in most cases appointed by the school administration), an assistant chair, a coordinator of the school counseling services, a media liaison, a staff notification coordinator, a communication coordinator, and a crowd management coordinator(s). Other team members can be assigned to sub-teams and take on specific roles and functions such as a security liaison, a medical liaison, evacuation and transport coordinator, etc. The committee must assign substitute team members so that their absence will not incapacitate the team. However, the desirability of including the many available individuals with valuable skills should be balanced by the need for a small, efficient, cohesive team (Lichtenstein et al., 1995). Optimally, a school crisis team comprises part of a set of system-wide crisis response teams that include a regional team (that also serves as liaison between state resources and regional needs) and a local district team (that also serves as liaison between regional services and the individual school-based crisis response team's needs). The community/state system must provide crisis teams with general training with respect to generic crisis intervention concepts, principles, policies, and practices. Selected representatives from the school system may be trained through contracts with selected specialists and collaborating agencies, such as universities, hospitals, and national mental health and education organizations. They may then, in turn, provide training to their colleagues. Additionally, each sub-team or designated specialist may require specialized assignment-related training.

Crisis Education, Simulations, and Drills

No crisis response plan can succeed well without the regular implementation of drills, readiness checks, school-wide simulations, and periodic tabletop drills. In interactive tabletop exercises, the crisis response team discusses how members would respond to various crisis situations, gleaning the manual protocols' strengths and gaps. Lessons learned from these should lead to adaptations in the existing procedures, or to the adoption of new ones.

Experience has shown that education of staff regarding children in disaster can meaningfully contribute to the effectiveness of crisis response in real time. School staff education should cover crisis theory; normal reactions to abnormal events; psychological needs of students, parents, and school staff in crisis; and how teachers can apply their instructional abilities to support their pupils and teach them positive coping skills at a time of crisis.

Educational and administrative staff as well as students should participate in school-wide drills that include rehearsing self-protection during and after a disaster (e.g., "duck and cover" for an earthquake), evacuation procedures, usage of intercom and cellular systems to permit school-wide and between-site communication despite telephone outages, and safe dissemination of students and personnel during rescue efforts (Nader & Pynoos, 1993).

Simulations can be written beforehand or added while the simulated event unfolds. Preparatory training that employed simulations proved valuable in changing attitudes and removing barriers during a real community emergency (Ayalon, 1998). Schools also benefited from a school-wide simulation of war conditions (Klingman, 1978, 1982), and students profited from a class-focused simulation of coping with death (Klingman, 1983, 1985a).

Altogether, the plan provides a general model and focuses on generic principles, but must be tailored to the particular school and to its specific needs and available resources. Moreover, its procedures must be flexible and undergo regular reevaluation at least annually and, when necessary, be modified. In this regard, core committee members should familiarize themselves not only with the types of natural or technological disasters possible in the school's particular geographical region but also with the potential deliberate human disasters that may strike during the given time period (e.g., anthrax threat, unsolved repeated shootings in the area). Committee members should also thoroughly review and analyze past mass crises and disaster response cases within their own school as well as other schools, in both minor and larger-scale events.

ANTICIPATORY INTERVENTION LEVEL

The anticipatory level of intervention refers to measures taken prior to an impending crisis/disaster that may have a detrimental effect on the target population or the school organization unless they undergo specific preparatory intervention. This level of intervention is not always present, because not all disasters have a warning phase that permits taking anticipatory measures; it is relevant for disasters that can be forecasted, such as some natural disasters or impending threats like war. Anticipatory disaster preparedness aims to prepare both organizationally and psychologically for various pre-identified contingencies using selective preventive measures (Mrazek & Haggerty, 1994). Such interventions target the school as an organization, the student body, and high-risk populations needing preparatory intervention (e.g., claustrophobic teachers who may need to stay in crowded shelters, asthmatic students who may need to use gas masks, students with behavior problems, students with special needs).

Organizationally, school-based anticipatory prevention is geared to review, reorganize, adjust, and modify the school system's crisis response plan protocols to meet the specific expected disaster-related conditions. Guidance, school-wide drills, and simulations must now relate to the more concrete, real-time information about the impending dangers. Simulations should be based first and foremost on systematic, accurate, and continuously updated information collection, and on its ongoing analysis and age-appropriate presentation breakdown. In addition, the crisis team should reexamine its coordination with community mental health and other community services. Time allowing, anticipatory prevention also encompasses studying and analyzing similar past events and interventions and their impact on the specific school and/or other schools, as well as rewriting manual scenarios (based on updated information and the analyses of past responses) for crisis team training and school-wide and class simulation exercises.

Psychoeducationally, anticipatory intervention aims to prepare students and staff to effectively cope with the impending stressors beforehand. The school-based anticipatory program provides specific preparatory information in order to desensitize students to stressful encounters, provide stress inoculation, and, when appropriate and possible, permit behavioral rehearsals prior to the stress point. Preparations must account for the fact that the bona fide, impending nature of the anticipatory activities may elicit extreme stress and thus should involve social support as well. The preparations for unconventional weapons prior to the two Gulf Wars in Israel demonstrate such anticipatory interventions. Prevention in this anticipatory period aimed to ensure children's familiarity and competence with gas masks and other protective measures against chemical fallout. The school-based intervention consisted of an educational phase; a skill-training phase that involved instructions and physical demonstrations of the protective equipment; and a few standardized training sessions based on gradual exposure. Through simulations of donning, learning to fasten, and breathing through the gas masks, pupils were expected to gain a sense of control. Trainers conveyed the expectation that students would thus withstand the threat of unconventional warfare effectively should it erupt.

Trainers also conveyed the expectation that students could help train siblings and older persons in the household as well as help them don the masks properly in real time; many children were reported to have been helpful in this regard during the 1991 Gulf War.

The case of parents who are about to leave home on combat missions is another illustration of children comprising a high-risk group requiring anticipatory intervention. The school can help children deal with the expected separation before departure as well as at the point of deployment. Deployment interrupts the natural family order and arouses anger, anxiety, and a sense of lack of control, which can be further intensified by rumors or media coverage. Anticipatory intervention can focus on factors influencing children's adjustment to parental absence, particularly explicit supportive communication that provides children with a clear, understandable rationale for the deployment (Figley, 1993).

The two levels described above comprise predisaster interventions. Next, we move to actual disaster response and intervention measures.

POSTDISASTER IMMEDIATE ORGANIZATIONAL RESPONSE LEVEL

When major disaster strikes, a school usually enters a state of organizational crisis. This disruption may physically affect the system as a whole and threaten its basic operational patterns. Simultaneously with the rescue efforts, strategic action must be taken to mitigate existing undesirable organizational developments, avoid further unnecessary ones, enlist and empower available resources, and optimally resolve associated problems as soon as possible under the new, real circumstances.

The organizational context is extremely important, if not crucial in the impact and immediate postdisaster phases. The initial response to disaster draws to a great extent from the efficacy of the predisaster crisis response plan and training, especially the trained activation of automatic reactions such as predesignated evacuation procedures to predesignated shelters. The first steps of crisis management after a disaster are often the most difficult because of the team's shock, concerns about the level of threat, time pressures, limited (or no) control, high uncertainty, and response-option constraints (Burnett, 1998). In our own work with schools following mass disaster, we have repeatedly witnessed unprepared schools neglecting many organizational intervention variables, often those very variables most critical for effective crisis management. (See Klingman, 1987 for a delineation of some organizational aspects of disaster response following a catastrophic school transportation accident.) Furthermore, disaster conditions rarely mimic a crisis response plan or theoretical model precisely, thus necessitating many on-the-spot alternations and modifications.

The following two steps can offer critical assistance in the impact and immediate postdisaster phase: rescue, on-site triage, and regaining of control should be initiated concurrently with initial organizational crisis management efforts.

Rescue, On-Site Triage, and Regaining a Sense of Control

Immediately after the disaster, the most urgent needs comprise direct, elementary, and concrete relief. These primary needs must take priority. In line with the school's crisis response plan, interventions must center first on logistical and practical actions: rescuing life, ensuring physical safety, providing emergency medical aid, supplying drinks to avoid dehydration and induce a calming effect by filling a basic familiar need, evacuating students in cases of structural damage or ongoing life threat, protecting students from unnecessary exposure to traumatic scenes, and helping restore a sense of order as much as possible.

Any psychosocial intervention at this time should be directed to serve these ends and ensure the sense of psychological safety, utilizing principles of mental health triage (i.e. determining the severity of need for each individual/group). The major tenet of triage upholds that in certain settings and under certain conditions it is not possible to provide help to everyone in need; thus, decisions must be based instead on the most efficient utilization of the limited known resources to best prevent the most harm. During a school disaster, this will first mean search and rescue, ensuring the physical safety of self and significant others, and then soothing and guidance. Attending to and resolving these more "practical" issues generally comprise a necessary precondition to an individual's or the school organization's capacity to benefit from early psychoeducational intervention. For example, injured students must be quickly transferred to medical facilities. To protect uninjured students from physical danger or unnecessary exposure to potentially traumatic scenes, relocation to safer areas on the school grounds or off campus may be in order. These logistical actions must precede any others.

Activation of simple practical measures can counteract the chaotic situations typifying large-scale disasters. Such activities include taking attendance, accounting for missing individuals, recording the hospital destination of injured children, controlling and recording the release of children to their parents. Technical failures in recording and monitoring the dissemination of children immediately following the event can exacerbate the stress response of both children and adults in the aftermath of trauma (Nader & Pynoos, 1993). School principals have described the search for the whereabouts of injured children or bodies dispersed to community or regional hospitals as an additional stressor in the immediate aftermath of a school disaster (Nader & Pynoos, 1993). This can be minimized by running orderly lists and pre-assigning personnel to support the parents during these critical moments. These personnel members must receive special preparation for the procedure of delivering bad news to parents.

Inasmuch as separation comprises a well-recognized source of children's stress, an important task consists of helping students who await reunification with their family members. In the immediate phase after disaster strikes, pupils may exhibit overwhelming anxiety about the whereabouts and safety of their loved ones (e.g., parents, siblings, close friends). During the waiting time, extremely anxious children may produce their own fantasies and related concerns of threat and injury to their loved ones. Nader and Pynoos (1993) noted that such fantasies might later become images that intrude into the child's life and may alter attachment behavior with family members and school personnel. Practical steps to connect students and staff with their families (e.g., by providing access to telephones) will offer emotional as well as functional support.

Initial Organizational Crisis Management

In general, the administrative intervention is geared toward the reactivation and revitalization of the school as a central, functioning community institution and support system. Concurrent with the rescue and triage operations described above, the first two essential steps toward organizational crisis management comprise the need to:

1. *Establish a command post and communication channels.* A critically important first step comprises calling in the crisis management team, relieving its members of any other tasks, and aiding them to set up a command post that includes a communication center. Two-way ongoing communication must be established with all concerned parties, both within the school and with outside agencies.

2. *Collect information and prioritize interventions.* The second step begins with the systematic collection of information. The team must sort out and properly identify the more relevant information to establish the overall crisis picture, to provide a basis for prioritizing further actions. Priorities derive from the simultaneous classification of strategies according to their threat level, time pressure, degree of control, and response-option constraints. Based on initial environmental analysis, the team should formulate situation-specific core tasks, evaluate strategic options, and actively predict the upcoming stage in the crisis. To maintain strategic control, these tasks and options should be kept tentative and require that the organization reconfigure itself through the deployment of human and material resources.

Helping the Helper and Caregiver

Mass disaster has a tremendous impact not only on victims and on community bystanders but also on helpers, including rescue workers, volunteers, and mental health professionals. Mitigating the helpers' stress is a vital component of intervention and should be organized as an early, on-site preventive process. Mental health professionals, as well as all others present on site (e.g., school administrators, teachers, rescue workers, volunteers), may be exposed to physical danger, and evidence violent death, mass death, and the death of children. Those who join the disaster scene may find it difficult to disassociate themselves from the ordeal.

The extreme anxiety, confusion, and pressure experienced by everyone present at the school are often directed at the mental health professional through a myriad of questions and urgent requests to help school administration, staff, parents, and students. Some of these requests are clearly outside the traditional role definition of the professional's activity, and it is frequently impossible to fulfill the overall level of expectations. Under such circumstances, it is quite a challenge for a mental health professional to be able to prioritize his or her actions, to define roles clearly, and to communicate in an organized and authoritative way with clients. Even when this is successfully achieved, the weight of pressing professional activities may be extremely demanding. Thus mental health professionals are at risk for experiencing extreme psyhological as well as physical fatigue. They are also at risk for overidentification with victims (i.e., compassion fatigue resulting in vicarious victimization). Children victims in particular evoke protective and nurturing feelings in most caregivers. Thus the situation demands that involved mental health professionals come to terms with and regulate their own reactions to the trauma before they can further help others, and that they psychologically "refuel" during their extensive involvement in trauma work. Interventions relevant to "helping the helpers" may therefore prove critical. Interventions to "help the helpers" should include both structuring of pragmatic 'technical' procedures and addressing situation-specific psychological needs. The technical procedures include working in pairs or mental health teams, organizing shifts and procedures for getting into and out of a scene, rotating personnel, providing a break area, teaching relaxation techniques, and the provision of on-the-spot group support. The psychological needs are met via group meetings around forms of debriefing (see the discussion of psychological debriefing later in this chapter).

The school personnel need some form of debriefing as well. Considering time pressure, this may be best delivered by using the team approach referred to as the pyramid procedure. A core of mental health workers form their own group (i.e., support system) to be debriefed and then, in turn, provide an adapted/modified debriefing to other helper groups (e.g., to school counselors) who, in turn, work with teachers.

PRIMARY PREVENTIVE INTERVENTION LEVEL

When safety is secured, primary prevention follows. The term primary prevention as used here refers to the measures and mental-health oriented interventions directed at the general school population that is under extreme stress but not yet experiencing maladjustment, via psychoeducational, social, and simple procedural, group, and interpersonal activities.

Central to the very concept of primary prevention in the context of a traumatic incident is timing. The generic principle of immediacy implies early intervention, before chronicity develops. Hence, clinicians, educators, and researchers have developed a rather large range of school-based primary prevention activities directed at pupils, staff, and families. We will briefly describe the primary organizational actions and elaborate more fully on a number of advisable primary psychoeducational measures to be implemented at this crucial time period in the schools.

When safety has been secured, psychoeducational action should follow, targeting students, teachers, parents, school administrators, support staff, and mental health personnel. As elaborated next, the early postdisaster period following the impact period requires several important psychoeducational actions at the primary prevention level: school-based briefings; establishment of a new routine via classroom crisis intervention; disaster-related rituals; support for students' funeral attendance; targeting student absenteeism; technological interventions (such as hotlines, internet, and computer-assisted trauma intervention); large-group parent intervention; solution-focused guidance; teachable moments and curricular adaptations; and adjustments of the roles of teachers and school mental health professionals. Note that the sequence of common primary prevention intervention issues and strategies presented herein does not claim to be strictly chronological. Each disaster is unique, and any school-based psychoeducational intervention should match the school's situation-specific needs.

School-Based Staff and Student Briefing

After reestablishing a sense of basic physical and psychological safety, the school's most important step comprises the restoration of a sense of order and control. This first entails briefing staff and students. Toward this end, teachers must enter their classrooms appearing to be relatively calm, informed about the factual events, and knowledgeable about and sensitive to trauma-generated behaviors and needs. However, teachers may feel overwhelmed and reluctant at first to assume the role of mental health mediators and may even attempt to avoid facing the students, thus necessitating teachers' empowerment. Our experience demonstrates that even a short group briefing for teachers held before entering the classroom, co-led by the school principal and the school mental health professional, generally suffices to enable most, if not all, affected teachers to calmly enter their classrooms and refrain from avoiding activities related to the trauma.

At a minimum, this short briefing includes the school principal's acknowledgement of the feelings associated with the critical incident and dissemination of accurate, updated, clear, and factual information on what has happened; which safety and recovery measures have already been or will be taken on and off campus; situation-specific administrative considerations and guidelines; and the school's plans for the rest of the day or the days to come. The school counselor or psychologist should supplement the principal's briefing by reviewing the most basic information about adults' and pupils' expected responses; providing simple instruction in basic generic mental health principles and specific ideas for conducting and handling a planned class session, which will enable children a chance to tell their stories and begin to process them; and assuring teachers of the approachability and availability of the school mental health professionals for ongoing consultation.

When the critical incident occurs off campus while school is in session, this staff briefing, however short, should be held between classes. In a case where the critical incident occurs off campus after school hours, a special training session or sessions should be organized for the staff, before they meet their students. In the Israeli school system, teachers usually arrive earlier than usual the next morning for the short briefing session.

A large-group briefing assembly for students may follow. Rather than focusing on emotional processing of the trauma, this assembly aims to provide factual information, counteract any misinformation, acknowledge the impact of the event, relay the measures taken by the school, and outline and explain expected behaviors and procedures to follow. We encourage a gentle authoritarian leadership by the chief administrator or the school principal for conducting the large-group briefing for students and staff. This meeting should promote the school personnel's and student body's confidence in the school's leadership and support, and should signal an expectation for regaining control. In scheduling students' briefing assemblies, dividing students by grade level allows the briefing to be tailored to developmental needs. In cases where many students exhibit extreme anxiety, the large group may be influenced by mass emotion and become more difficult to control and should therefore be kept short, focusing on factual information and the administration's immediate plans. Experience has shown that a better alternative in situations of extremely heightened emotionality is for the principal to go into each classroom separately to brief the students.

A supplementary extended meeting takes place later on, after school hours. The latter may serve to combine an expanded briefing and a psychoeducational intervention with a school mental health professional as co-leader. In this after-school group meeting, teachers should be encouraged to share their classroom experiences, report on students' reactions and coping strategies, describe class trauma-related activities, and further discuss their concerns. Beyond enabling some ventilation, this meeting helps teachers promote cognitive organization and self-control; set realistic expectations of themselves and their students; identify, recognize, and mobilize internal and external resources for their clinical mediating role; and restore self-resourcefulness. We found it beneficial to encourage the teachers to share in the group how they deal with their own children at home in times of crisis; or if they are not parents to use their past personal or professional experience as resources in a time of extreme crisis or stress. This discussion helps teachers recognize their ability to "do a good job," learn from each other, reduce their sense of helplessness, recover self-esteem, regain control over resources and objectives, and resume their sense of personal and professional responsibility. This process of teachers' empowerment was presented in detail by Wolmer, Laor, and Yazgan (2003), and a similar process with school counselors was described by Klingman (2002c).

The most exposed or affected teachers may need a separate meeting for a short psychological debriefing procedure (see below). The authors' and other Israeli practitioners' experience indicates that the hardest-hit teachers benefit from participating in some kind of debriefing that allows them to process and restructure their personal traumatic experience (Wolmer et al., 2003).

The Establishment of a New Routine: Psychoeducational Classroom Crisis Intervention

In line with the generic intervention principles of immediacy and proximity (see Chapter 9), the importance of a return to familiar and predictable school routines as quickly as possible cannot be overemphasized. The return to routine despite upheaval reestablishes a sense of order and reassures children that the once stable, although presently shaken world is already on its way to recovery. Returning to a Lower Manhattan high school after the September 11 attack, one student commented, "Outside everything changed, but inside the school everything felt the same; it feels like escaping from the world" (*The New York Times*, October 10, 2001). Another informal observation by teachers following the Hurricane Andrew disaster highlights the value of school routine. Teachers reported that some students did not want to return home after school because things felt normal at school, whereas they still encountered considerable hurricane destruction at home and in their neighborhood (Vernberg, 2002). Prinstein, La Greca, Vernberg, and Silverman (1996) found that children who reported high levels of assistance from parents, friends, and teachers in resuming their normal roles and routines during the first few months after Hurricane Andrew reported significantly fewer PTSD symptoms 7 months later. However, this routine must not be equated with "business as usual."

At least in the short-run, some aspects of the environment are not "as usual" or "as they used to be." Moreover, extreme material and psychological changes resulting from disasters, such as the loss of loved ones or of a home, may never be wiped away or reversed (Gist & Lubin, 1999). Thus, the process of fully returning to organizational as well as personal predisaster functioning necessitates a period of adjustment referred to as "newly defined normalcy" (Nader, 2001), or as exercising a *new routine*.

New routine refers to adaptations to the new circumstances and learning to live and function while embracing conflicting states of being. Following a disaster, teachers can guide children to acknowledge the possible co-existence of pain together with hopefulness and realize that both anxiety and satisfaction, or even some fun, do coexist.

Upon returning to the classroom after a disaster, the teacher must guide children in the new routine through the implementation of a teacher-mediated psychoeducational classroom crisis intervention. Teachers thus serve as clinical mediators. In many cases, the school staff may be the first to hear children's comprehensive account of the event as experienced by them and, also, the first to enable them to express and discuss their feelings and thoughts in a structured way within a safe environment. Wolmer et al. (2003) examined the role of teachers as clinical mediators and discussed the rationale for classroom-activated, teacher-mediated interventions. They asserted that practical considerations (e.g., cost effectiveness, limited resources, and the reluctance of most victims to seek professional help) and conceptual motives (e.g., "normalization") mandate that disaster relief efforts involve as many children as possible, by working with them in groups rather than as individuals. Most teachers already share intimate, trustful, long-lasting relationships with students and their parents and are ready to take on some therapeutic role. They also have numerous opportunities to closely observe and follow-up students in their natural setting. Some teachers today may even be experienced with preventive interventions that were previously incorporated into the regular curriculum, such as violence prevention. Others may require more comprehensive preparation for their role in leading a classroom crisis intervention at the preparedness level, and more support of the mental health team in its implementation.

In the teacher-mediated crisis intervention, the teacher must affirm students' safety and then create a friendly, calming classroom milieu. The teacher achieves this milieu by communicating accepting, nonjudgmental, empathic, and caring concern, and by conveying assurance, reassurance, and structure. The crisis intervention contains several components: information provision, emotional and cognitive processing, creative exploration of personal meaning, and practical assistance.

Information

In the first major step in classroom crisis intervention, the teacher must provide the students with information as to what happened, what actions are being carried out to ensure the safety of the students on campus and the safety of significant others off campus (e.g., parents, siblings, other family members, peers), and what is being done to prevent further adversities. Presenting, discussing, and clarifying what the adults around them are doing to restore safety and protection may be even as simple as informing them of tightened school and neighborhood security, or explaining the role and activity of the recovery forces and emergency services. Such facts help students view the event in a wider perspective and achieve some level of desensitization toward reminders of the traumatic event. Information should be accurate, updated, clear, and simple, tailored to the students' level of conceptual understanding, and devoid of clichés or euphemisms. Part and parcel with the provision of information, the teacher must correct misinformation and misperceptions as well as define or redefine concepts and terms (e.g., related to terrorism or biochemical warfare).

Emotional and Cognitive Processing

Students may also require the teacher to help them process and interpret their observations, thoughts, and feelings about what they experienced, heard, saw on TV, and read. Considering the wide differences in children's willingness to disclose thoughts and feelings in the classroom setting, we recommend providing an opportunity for the ventilation of feelings but not insisting on it. Thus, it is not advisable to seat participants in a circle and ask each how he or she feels (Kenardy et al., 1996; Scott, 1998), students should feel genuinely free to engage or disengage. Moreover, we suggest a careful and limited inquiry about feelings, so as to avoid sensitizing and inducing a sense of vulnerability. An emphasis should be placed on moving back early from a predominantly emotional processing level toward a cognitive processing level. The emphasis then shifts to "depathologization" of the physical, emotional, mental, and behavioral reactions and symptoms that are already or may soon be experienced, thus providing reassurance and mitigating worry. Teachers must accept, validate, and normalize all reactions. Considering these limitations, the initial processing of the traumatic event during the first class meeting may include questions along the following general sequence:

- *Fact gathering* (Where were you when it happened? What did you first see, hear, sense? What actually happened?)
- *Thoughts* (What were your first thoughts? How have they changed? What are your thoughts now?)

- *Behavioral reactions* (What was your initial reaction? What course of action did you take then?)
- *Feelings* (What do you remember about your immediate feelings? How have they changed? How do you feel now?)
- *Observed happenings and behavioral reactions of others* (How did your family members react? Your friends? Your neighbors?)

Information about expected symptoms can provide vast reassurance to students, enable them to categorize their own reactions as "normal coping in adverse situations," and prevent secondary symptoms such as worries over bodily or psychic reactions (Brom & Kleber, 1989).

Creative Exploration of Personal Meaning

Next, this first classroom session provides a thoroughly apt setting for each student to explore the personal meaning of the tragic event via a series of expressive, semi-structured, verbal and nonverbal activities as described in Chapter 12.

Practical Assistance

The first class session should end by offering the option of practical help and support through a description of available school and community support services. The teacher can also provide very simple situation-specific practical coping suggestions such as safety measures, danger avoidance behaviors, and deep breathing relaxation techniques. The teacher may review skills (e.g. for reducing stress and managing anxiety) that may have been taught during crisis education in the predisaster period. He or she may further encourage and facilitate the process of students' learning from each other useful situation-specific adaptive methods to handle fears and helplessness. This may increase the students' ability to tolerate and manage symptoms rather than resorting to self-defeating behavior.

Brock (2002a, 2002b) devised a school-based, classroom-activated, teacher-led crisis intervention model to foster psychological closure for schoolchildren who were neither directly involved nor severely traumatized by a critical incident. The six steps in this model comprise: (a) acknowledging the event and its effect and explaining the session's purpose; (b) providing facts and dispelling rumors to foster students' reality-based understanding of the event; (c) sharing stories to enhance students' sense of connectedness with classmates; (d) sharing reactions to normalize them; (e) empowering students to regain a sense of control, including brainstorming strategies to prevent the event's reoccurrence, discussing coping options, and reviewing tales of heroism and survival; and (f) engaging students in situation-specific age-appropriate activities, such as preparation for attending or participating in funerals or for creative memorial projects. In carrying out this intervention, which may range from 1 to 3 hours, the teacher consults with the school counselor or psychologist, and tailors it to the students' developmental level. Additional preventive interventions may be necessary later, for the whole class if such an intervention is conducted during relatively chaotic circumstances, or for specific students who are not ready yet to face the emotions brought on by discussing the trauma.

Disaster-Related Rituals

The need for ritual intensifies when a school faces trauma. If no rituals are readily available or in place, students may spontaneously create "new" ones (Klingman & Shalev, 2001; Klingman, Shalev, & Pearlman, 2000). In mass trauma situations, rituals often occur in a chronological sequence: spontaneous, unplanned expressions in the first hours or days, followed by funerals, then official memorial services and anniversary events (Eyre, 1999). Spontaneous, initial, informal, "popular" rituals often begin within hours of a disaster. These typically include visiting the disaster site or other significant sites associated with the critical incident or the deceased, as well as gathering in places of worship. Visitors lay down flowers, toys, or other mementoes, light candles, and pen the names of lost classmates or others on the walls as well as messages expressing personal and communal grief and other emotions and thoughts. Candlelight vigils provide spiritual strength while waiting for victims' rescue or recovery. Some may feel the urge to do "something" such as donating blood and collecting funds. Religious-based rituals such as nondenominational school assemblies, funerals, memorials, or composed prayers allow children to participate in a structured concrete farewell from lost significant others (see Chapter 12). Such therapeutic rituals contribute substantially to children's grief management (Dyregrov, 1996). These gatherings can serve as large-group supportive environments in which students and staff connect, communicate, receive guidance, and feel active as they share, donate, volunteer, and join together physically and emotionally.

In certain cases, a careful and sensitive school staff may need to channel or supervise a spontaneously created ritual, while still allowing it. Attention to this phenomenon is important because these rituals hold significant implications for trauma management in terms of logistical and psychological immediate post-impact recovery. For example, we were consulted by a high school PTA about a ritual that students developed after their classmate's dead body was found in a small grove in the school's neighborhood. The students began gathering every night in that grove, lighting a fire, and "hanging out" there together. Parents and school personnel felt concerned about the morbid as well as safety aspects of this ritual. Our collaborative consultation clarified that this ritual served both as a fear-defying activity and to unite the students for social support. The school administration and parents decided to continue allowing the ritual but with additional security measures to be provided by the parents and local security personnel who would patrol the grove from a slight distance.

Planned rituals and anniversaries must be carefully and sensitively designed and monitored. These planned memorial events hold significance in that they mark a physical as well as social time, thereby enabling collective remembrance and the expression of a school memory. During their annual Remembrance Day ceremony, many schools in Israel commemorate the entire list of fallen soldiers and terrorist victims from all alumni families over the years. This creates a supportive community for the bereaved families in the school that their child attended; concomitantly, this ceremony demonstrates to the current school population the deep personal ties of the school with its students.

However, memorial ceremonies and first anniversaries can be a fragile time. School staff must be aware and prepared for the triggering of emotional reactions and symptoms by any first postdisaster memorial ceremony, especially the one conducted very close in time to, or at the site of the traumatic incident.

Support for Students' Funeral Attendance

Children's attendance of the funerals of loved ones, classmates, or teachers comprises a frequent issue encountered following school disaster and requiring primary preventive psychoeducational intervention, through in-class discussions with teachers. Adults, especially parents, often tend to shield children from the funeral experience, thinking it too difficult for children to endure. Indeed, teachers and parents can advise students of the many ways to depart from the deceased other than a funeral. In-class discussions can generate alternative creative rituals to be conducted at the school while the formal funeral is in progress (see below).

However, barring children who wish to attend a funeral from doing so may create an environment that denies them a sense of actively participating in the grieving process, enhances denial, and encourages avoidance. Moreover, some children who are denied this opportunity may construct fantasies of what occurs during these ceremonies that may be more frightening than the reality, and they may also feel left out of an important collective ritual (Schonfeld, 1993). The funeral ritual may enable the child to begin the process of departing from the deceased and of sharing grief with significant others. Furthermore, it may model for the child how people comfort one another, mourn, and honor the dead. Thus, we recommend that students be allowed the opportunity to attend if they wish. However, because of the stress involved, the school should accentuate, first, the advisability of inviting a significant adult to accompany them during the funeral and, second, the legitimacy of keeping at a distance and of leaving with this adult at any point during the ceremony. The teacher should also provide simple, age-appropriate information about any anticipated customs such as an open casket viewing or gravesite ceremony. The school should also make provision for some school staff, such as homeroom teachers, the school nurse, and a school counselor, to be present at the funeral(s) to monitor students' reactions and attend to their affective responses. Reports gathered from 90 parents, 10 days after a terrorist incident killing three students from a junior high school in Jerusalem, showed parents viewed their children's attendance of their fellow students' funerals as a significant and helpful experience in coping with the event (Cohen, 2000).

Targeting Student Absenteeism

Students' immediate return to school and class attendance following a disaster may comprise a critical stage in first-order preventive intervention. Some students may be absent due to injury, hospitalization and medical check-ups, or because of practical problems such as transportation difficulties or evacuation to other areas. Other students may be absent because their families are coping with practical daily survival, like in cases where the family home was badly damaged. Some students may remain at home due to their parents' anxiety or their own avoidance behavior such as that resulting from fears to board a school bus after a mass school bus accident or a terrorist bus bombing, or because of survivor guilt feelings (e.g., Klingman, 2001b). Outreach to absent students and their families requires the coordinated efforts of peers, teachers, and, when needed, a school counselor, school social worker, or truancy officer in prolonged absentee cases. Students identified as psychologically resistant to returning to school should be proactively approached and encouraged to do so; those who persist in their avoidant behavior should be referred to professional consultation or treatment. Whenever possible and appropriate, the school can activate peers both in encouraging the absentee to return to school and in easing the student's return; this role simultaneously serves as a task-oriented adaptive coping experience for the peers.

Flexibility and often creativity in meeting situation-specific needs, especially of children who find it difficult to remain in the classroom and follow the school routine, should be encouraged. Students who wish to be excused from class to see a counselor may receive a pass to the counseling center. The school may also offer alternative ad hoc support frameworks to students who find it difficult to remain in class. This entails making available a *safe room* or a *safe area* to which students can be referred for relaxation, comfort, or support. School staff members may operate these safe areas, with the occasional visit by the school counselor to touch base with students if they need additional support. For example, following a junior high school mass transportation disaster, external mental health workers and the school counselor collaborated to locate a room in the school to accommodate a few extremely anxious students who could not return to their classrooms and who were selectively withholding speech (Klingman, 1987; Klingman, Koenigsfeld, & Markman, 1987). Some students came to this ad hoc art, activity, and creativity room at the suggestion of mental health staff members working with them; others joined after hearing about its open-door policy from their homeroom teachers. The creativity room facilitated individual and group activities such as helping establish a school memorial corner. Such activities may provide students with a release for strong emotions and with a positive outlet for their energy while responding to their immediate psychological needs.

Technological Interventions: Hotlines, Internet, and Computer-Assisted Trauma Intervention

The use of so-called modern technology in general, and computer-based technologies in particular, may hold the potential to impact trauma preventive intervention; given the rapid advances in technology, this potential will increase. Despite its limitations and disadvantages (Klingman, 1996), technology furnishes a practical means for outreach when face-to-face contact is not feasible. Members of the school community who are housebound due to injury or travel restrictions during a state of emergency, or who feel they cannot benefit from the generic intervention, can easily call in to hotlines. The Internet and other telecommunication means provide large-scale information dissemination and serve as alternative support systems. Students can also participate in computer-based interventions.

Telephone Hotlines. In a large-scale school disaster, the school can set up school-based emergency telephone hotlines for the students, parents, and staff (Klingman, 1987, 2002b). Because the hotline is operated in school and by school and school-linked personnel such as the school psychologist or counselor or affiliated mental health professionals, it usually remains stigma free, unlike the case with mental health centers. Such hotlines involve active listening, soothing responses, correcting misinformation, behavioral guidance, and at times, simple anxiety-reduction techniques. Teachers may obtain advice about their students' situation-specific problems, suggestions concerning handling the class, and guidance in adapting lesson contents to the circumstances (Klingman, 1996, 2002a, 2002b; Raviv, 1993).

Fiber Optics and Communication Satellites. In the immediate wake of a large-scale disaster, information needs to be disseminated quickly, easily, and effectively. The Internet enables retrieval of information as well as communication. If available, broadband Internet access can provide a unique solution in cases of overload or temporary collapse of the school's electronic information technology (e.g., portable cellular equipment, telephones, facsimile lines) immediately after a disaster. The school website can post information about pupils' safety, evacuation arrangements, and other situation-specific procedures. Two-way e-mail communication can facilitate logistics such as a specific parent's arrangement for a child's pick-up. The school may prioritize e-mail messages according to risk, for immediate or later response.

The Internet permits both school-based and home-based rapid access to vast amounts of expert information. The school can screen and control official authorities' information bulletins, translating them into age-appropriate language for the students. Immediate or same-day information about stress reactions and the best ways to handle these responses (possibly composed during the predisaster period) can be posted on computer bulletin boards targeting concerned pupils, parents, and teachers.

During school closure, school staff may communicate with pupils by electronic mail, or develop their own website to assist pupils in managing stress. Recently developed technologies may add video and interactive components to enable some kinds of supportive counseling (for a discussion of the potentials in healing in the technological era, see Bennett, 2001). Internet communities, or "wired neighborhoods," make it possible for children to interact amongst themselves without leaving home or shelter. Mental health personnel can also use the e-mail for professional collaboration and consultation with geographically removed experts.

Additionally, virtual video games allow children to use screen graphics and construct a character and environment of their own choice and then experience through play the control of this virtual environment. This outlet may serve as a possible escape valve for anxiety and anger.

Computer-Assisted Trauma Intervention. Kronik, Akhmerov, and Speckhard (1999) introduced a computer-assisted intervention model for disaster victims. This computer-based, psychologist-assisted, interactive psychological software program was developed as diagnostic and intervention technology for addressing the posttraumatic responses of adolescent victims of the Chernobyl disaster. The program, called LifeLine, plays a remedial function in that it offers adolescent victims new ways in which to experience time (personal, past, present, and future). Kronik et al. developed the program to assist middle- and high-school students incorporate an overwhelmingly traumatic event into their life narrative, to address shattered world assumptions, and to rebuild a more positive life orientation. Schools can develop and creatively implement tools such as LifeLine at relatively little cost.

Large-Group Parent Interventions

In the aftermath of disaster, schools frequently employ a large-group assembly as a preventive intervention to brief parents in the school auditorium after school hours. As elaborated in detail in Chapter 13, the assembly can offer a problem-centered organizational, psychoeducational, and social intervention. Such an assembly may follow the 4-phase crisis management briefing intervention mode described below in the section on psychological debriefing (Everly, 2000b). Such a debriefing brings together a group of up to 300 individuals, requires about an hour to conduct, and includes a breakdown into small-group meetings.

Solution-Focused Class Guidance

In the aftermath of a traumatic event, a natural preoccupation emerges with fear, stress, anxiety symptoms, and problems (Solomon, 1995). When coupled with mental health professionals' emphasis on emotional expression, the school may often neglect alternative, active means of coping and messages of strength and resilience. One school-based intervention aiming to counteract this climate, solution-focused guidance, hones in on positive, active solutions.

Solution-focused guidance (SFG) can serve as a basis for class or group discussion that aims to empower students to use their own resources in practical ways to confront an aversive experience. Klingman (2002c) found empirical evidence for the effectiveness of conducting SFG with school counselors during a nationwide political trauma – the recent Palestinian uprising in Israel. Additional informal evaluations have shown that well trained counselors and teachers can successfully use SFG, with some modifications, as a class discussion tool with high school students following terrorist attacks.

SFG emphasizes a gradual shift from "problem-talk" to "solution-talk," and eventually toward a future-oriented pictorial plan for life without the undesired problems. The discussion moves from emotional expression of the adverse experience, problem, or threat appraisal, to a focus of attention on positive aspects (e.g., courageous acts), strengths, and active coping. Assuming that people successfully solve everyday problems, the intervention empowers participants to focus on, recognize, and use these inner resources. Drawing on the solution-focused therapeutic approach for children (Selekman, 1997), SFG underscores mottoes like enhancing small changes in mental outlook, looking for small changes to bring about bigger changes, continuing what works and stopping what does not, and fixing only what is broken. Normalization and reframing are central. To achieve reframing, participants are guided to look for alternative, different, or new interpretations and descriptions of events and the resulting emotional, cognitive, and behavioral reactions. Corresponding with the narrative approach, SFG enables participants to tell their own story so as to make sense of chaos, distill and discover a trajectory in life, and view life with a sense of agency rather than victimization (Seligman, 2002). Discussion progresses to rebuild confidence, rediscover a belief that some things can improve, and invest in self-efficacy. As these abilities improve, the facilitator can shift from the roles of expert advice-giver and technical guide to a more facilitating role. As can be seen, SFG derives flexibly from several models of social and individual psychology and borrows various techniques from other therapeutic approaches, yet retains its own theoretical integrity.

Teachable Moments and Curricular Adaptations

Two kinds of teacher-mediated interventions appear to be useful: (a) the aforementioned classroom crisis intervention that focuses on directly discussing the traumatic event with students and attempts to enhance processing of the traumatic experience as a first-aid psychosocial intervention; and (b) a later intervention concerning the selection and utilization of curricular subject matter that can indirectly help students process the trauma, using rational and emotional processing, and a range of adjustments to standard curricula, as described below.

Teachers recognize that after a disaster they must adapt lesson plans to meet students' needs rather than merely covering regular curricula. A "teachable moment" refers to the time when students are most curious and eager to learn because they are able and psychologically motivated to apply this learning at that specific time. Practically, this infers teaching a subject matter when student interest level reaches its peak. The intensity of disastrous events provides many such teachable moments. For example, students can be invited to explore topics such as the causes and consequences of natural and human adversities while studying geography, ecology, social studies, and life skills. Our experience suggests that creative adaptations in the curriculum can tap the potential inherent in a teachable moment, by responding to students' interest and needs while enriching the educational program.

The best means to systematically implement educational interventions that respond to students' needs after disaster comprises a planned curriculum administered by classroom teachers with the ongoing consultation of mental health professionals. For optimal results, we recommend a coordinated approach that integrates the many areas of the regular curriculum as well as extracurricular activities that can incorporate aspects of the traumatic event. For example, in the aftermath of a terrorist attack, a language class may focus on essays about terrorism, justice, violence, safety, prejudice, and freedom, with students' papers becoming the springboard for class discussions. Also, the language teacher should address event-relevant vocabulary (e.g., debris, eradicate, fundamentalist). In a history class, issues concerning various nationalities in the Middle East can be explored. The American history teacher could teach the class about past responses to terror; various world leaders' verbal responses to the current attack ("the power of words"); and concepts such as fundamentalism, coalition, and culture war. The profile of negative, immoral leaders can be studied. The geography teacher can ask students to explore or create maps of Manhattan or Afghanistan, labeling strategic locations cited in newspaper articles. A journalism class may encourage the construction of a photo-journal composed of students' photography, newspaper photos, or pictures from websites. Science class can relate to biological and chemical weapons and their effects on the population, learning about precautions and protection measures.

Lesson plans can be geared to embrace many of the mental health aspects and principles presented in this book. For example, in order to confront fears, students in the language arts or fine arts classes could explore their own fears and then reverse the scenario and consider how the objects of their fears may, in turn, also be afraid of them. They could then move to creating booklets to help younger students do the same. In art class, students could explore their experience nonverbally (see also Chapter 12). The health class teacher can invite a mental health professional and use peer counselors to normalize feelings.

The education section of *The New York Times* presents lesson plans for schools around a central news article or essay that employs an interdisciplinary approach by grade level. These plans were developed in partnership with the Bank Street College of Education in New York City. Their advantage lies in their timely publication, often within hours of a tragic event, and their accessibility online for download from the Internet [http://nytimes.com/learning]. The U.S. Federal Emergency Management Agency (FEMA), American Red Cross, Vietnam Veterans of America Foundations, and others also often publish ideas for lesson plans and activities by grade level online following mass disasters.

Adjustments to the School Mental Health Professionals' Roles

A disaster creates unusual management issues for both school administration and the teaching staff, who require support and guidance. School administrators and the educational staff, beyond struggling with managing a relatively chaotic situation both organizationally and psychologically, may have to struggle with their own personal and possibly familial distress. Therefore, the mental health professionals should aim first and foremost to relieve some of the staff members' own emotional distress through consultations and group debriefings (Gordon et al., 1999).

The school mental health professionals, as consultants, must further offer help to both the administrative and educational staff in a variety of possible emergency school-based roles focusing on children's welfare at the immediate post-impact period. A major task comprises managing and coordinating all school-based mental-health focused interventions, integrating them into a whole school-based emergency organizational process, and ensuring that any school-based organizational decision-making takes mental health considerations into account. For example, the mental health professional must ensure that triage and risk screening are being well coordinated and supervised in line with the generic principles and based on a situation-specific triage and screening. This means that the crisis team's mental health coordinator also assumes *a supervisory role*. In this regard, the mental health coordinator should be careful to respect the lines of authority for decision-making, and the formal and hierarchical structure of the organization, inasmuch as school personnel may perceive this surrogate leadership position as a threat to the designated school leadership.

Organization-focused consultation involves assisting with mental health information relevant to organizational decision-making. The focus of consultation lies on reestablishing and facilitating the natural resources and support systems and networks as immediately as possible. The mental health professional points out to the school administration those psychologically relevant needs that have arisen because of the school organizational changes. He or she helps school staff to reassume their roles, empowering them by providing them with ideas and tools to do so under the new circumstances. Taking on roles of mediator, translator, and facilitator, the mental health professional indicates to them how to adapt clinically based protocols to the non-clinical settings (e.g., classrooms, school offices) regarding contents, procedures, and didactics and supports them to modify their responsibility to postdisaster conditions (Klingman, 2002b; Laor, Wolmer, Spirman & Weiner, 2003; Wolmer et al., 2003).

All these roles may necessitate a temporary departure from the usually practiced consultation mode. Given the reality of the disaster situation, the mental health professional must take a proactive-directive approach such as the *coercive-directive consultation approach* (Gutkin, 1999) that works best immediately after a traumatic incident. This approach refers to consultation regarding the immediate acute issues for which unilateral rather than shared consultation (as in the collaborative-directive approach) is the method of choice. The school counselor role as consultant, for example, should involve encouraging teachers to use their educational and teaching experience to address children's coping using curricular materials adapted to the situation. This may entail suggesting, and often showing, teachers what to teach and how to adapt their lesson plans. Moreover, because of the fluidity of the situation, mental health consultants must often rely primarily on their own judgment when recommending steps to be taken, or when selecting among intervention strategy options. The coercive-directive approach alone, however, does not suffice. The mental health professional should also incorporate systemic ecological thinking (Gutkin & Curtis, 1999), which attends both to the proximal (i.e., immediate antecedents and consequences) and the distal environmental variables (e.g., teachers' tolerance for pupils' acute stress response, parents' concerns for their child's safety) that may greatly impact children's responses and recovery. Whereas consultation is definitely directive and behavioral at first, later on in the school recovery process the consultant might consider shifting between consultation modes as necessary for different problems, until circumstances allow for a return to the preferred predisaster approach.

Because of the intense feelings of urgency, the school staff may expect the mental health professional not only to be knowledgeable in crisis intervention principles, but also to become actively involved in the problem-solving process when problems arise. We maintain that school-based disaster interventions by the mental health professionals should usually be as indirect as possible, bolstering natural support systems rather than displacing them. Thus, it is essential that the mental health consultant work closely with the school principal or one of the principal's assistants, who can coordinate the implementation of the consultant's input (Nader & Pynoos, 1991).

EARLY SECONDARY PREVENTIVE INTERVENTION LEVEL

Early secondary preventive intervention involves monitoring stress reactions early in the aftermath of a disaster. This intervention level consists of systematic school-wide outreach aimed at mass screening, early diagnosis, and case finding. Such interventions begin after the initial chaos has subsided and simultaneously with the aforementioned primary prevention activities, which are well under way.

The school offers a natural site for early monitoring of children and adolescents' behavior. Systematic screening of pupils, teaching staff, support staff, and administrators aims to identify acute cases showing early signs of behavioral and emotional adjustment difficulties and problems (e.g., those who are not responding to the generic primary prevention measures). Parents' needs should also be considered, as outlined in detail in Chapter 13. Charting a graphic representation of at risk-groups as a reference has demonstrated benefit in schools' attempts to establish priorities and divide labor accordingly (e.g., Klingman, 1987, 1996; Pynoos & Nader, 1988).

Figure 1 offers a graph illustrating concentric circles of risk, with the central point representing the primary victim(s). The names of individuals or groups of students or staff, or off-campus at-risk populations (e.g., siblings who attend other schools) should be plotted on the circles according to (a) intensity of exposure and (b) risk factors like previous loss, emotional and physical proximity to the primary victim, grief, and their interplay. Outreach may then be organized to approach those most affected first. This graph can be used in earlier stages of intervention and even be posted on the wall of the command post (Klingman, 1987). The graph maintains awareness among the mental health intervention team members of the actual and potential target groups and problems; enables a clear, detailed,

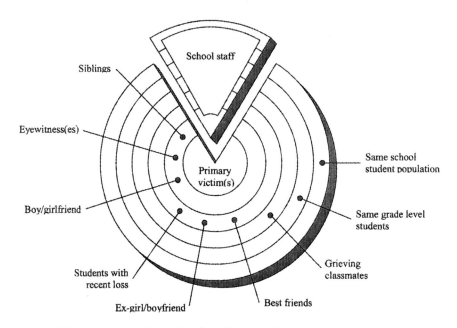

Figure. 1. Concentric circles of at-risk targets for outreach: An example.

and overall layout of the full scope of the intervention; promotes informed, systematic decision-making; fosters appropriate division of professional labor in accordance with priorities, expertise, and prior experience; and facilitates monitoring and feedback concerning the outreach efforts' efficacy.

Other early secondary preventive measures may include opening in-school ad hoc walk-in clinics and following up on telephone hotline callers and absent students. Once identified, primary victims are proactively approached for psychological first-aid that includes initiating sensitive psychological contact, exploring with them the dimension of the traumatic event, assisting them in taking concrete actions, and following up to evaluate progress (Slaikeu, 1984).

INDICATED SECONDARY PREVENTIVE INTERVENTION LEVEL

Indicated preventive interventions target only high-risk individuals who are identified as having detected markers or symptoms foreshadowing a *DSM-IV* (American Psychiatric Association, 1994) psychological disorder, but whose symptoms are not yet sufficiently severe to merit a full diagnosis at the current time. Thus, at this level of intervention, once immediate needs are not met through early secondary intervention measures, more established screening and help-giving patterns take over.

During the recovery phase, individuals who begin to show early symptoms of a disorder may become candidates for an indicated preventive intervention program designed to avert the full-blown manifestation of the disorder through more intensive and focused preventive strategies. Generally, these interventions aim at bringing the maladjustment under control rapidly, primarily to keep its impact minimal, reduce the duration of early symptoms, and halt its progression of severity. An additional aim comprises furnishing longer-term support to afflicted individuals and their families. The underlying expectation is that successful intervention during the early development of problems can prevent the occurrence of later, more serious dysfunction (Klingman, 2001b).

Whereas interventions at the preparedness, anticipatory, primary, and early secondary levels focus on generic principles, indicated intervention focuses more on intrapsychic and interpersonal processes. Rather than targeting the whole population, indicated intervention relates more to the unique needs of individuals, or of individuals in the small group when employing group counseling. This level of intervention aims to alleviate specific symptoms and to restore individual pre-crisis level of functioning. Indicated intervention in the school setting mostly takes the form of group counseling but differs from that of community-based clinics in two major ways. First, the school setting helps avoid stigmatization; educators themselves may also be involved in complementary school-based interventions. Second, indicated intervention in schools offers the advantage of daily contact with the pupils' educators, which opens a two-way flow of information about the pupils' needs and progress. Beyond apprising mental health professionals of how the pupil is coping in the natural environment, this communication flow facilitates teachers' ability to conduct activities that help the pupil through the crisis.

One form of indicated intervention most commonly used in the aftermath of traumatic events is psychological debriefing, a crisis intervention designed to relieve acute distress as well as to prevent further trauma-related distress for those individuals experiencing acute stress reactions.

Psychological Debriefing

Psychological debriefing (PD) after a traumatic event comprises a proactive semi-structured intervention approach designed to relieve event-related distress in normal people experiencing abnormally stressful circumstances. Most mental health agencies consider PD, conducted by an experienced, trained professional, to be the standard of care in large-scale disasters. Although PD can be used individually, it was originally designed as a group-format exposure procedure where participants share their detailed accounts of the trauma during a single session held within a few days of the event. Individual storytelling enables people to establish a coherent narrative of the event by pooling facts and highlighting predictable and manageable features, thereby helping survivors move on to a more confident outlook and set an agenda for recovery (Hodgkinson, 2000). Although ventilation of feelings constitutes a potentially important ingredient, the PD process focuses not on stimulation of emotions but predominantly on social, educative, and cognitive techniques, with an emphasis on resilience. The educative components help participants understand the incident's significance, sort out post-event psychological reactions, and normalize stress reactions through sharing. Cognitive techniques foster restructuring of distorted beliefs, mobilization of resources (e.g., group solidarity, sources of support), and preparation for likely future difficulties.

Mitchell (1983) developed the widely employed *Critical Incident Stress Debriefing (CISD)* approach. This formalized structured method calls for a single group meeting commonly conducted 2 to 14 days after a critical incident, lasting up to 3 hours, and comprising a highly standardized 7-phase discussion of the traumatic incident: introduction; fact-finding; exploration of the cognitions experienced; identification and expression of emotional reactions; acknowledgement of post-incident cognitive, somatic, emotional, and behavioral signs of distress; psychoeducation about stress and self-care; and facilitation of referrals and of returning to everyday life (Everly & Mitchell, 2000; Mitchell & Everly, 1997). In general, CISD aims to facilitate processes of psychological reconstruction and closure. When closure is not possible, CISD serves as a psychological triage mechanism to identify those in need of further care. Despite CISD's widespread use, its unique effectiveness in preventing PTSD remains ambiguous, requiring further empirical study. In the wake of mass trauma, group-format debriefing seems to be well received by participants and thus considered to be a beneficial means for community social education and outreach to a large population. However, researchers have recently called attention to findings showing that while some forms of formal PD may be helpful, some may be somewhat harmful for some people, while others may have no effect (Carlier, 2000; Everly & Mitchell, 2000; Mayou, Ehlers, & Hobbs, 2000).

Originally developed solely for use with emergency response personnel, over the years PD methods have been expanded for use with both responders and adult victims. However, only a few forms of PD were conducted with children and adolescents following mass traumas (e.g., Johnson, 1989; Klingman, 1987; Yule, 1992). In Yule's controlled study, debriefed children scored lower on intrusion and on unrelated fears than did non-debriefed children, but no differences emerged for avoidance, anxiety, or related fears. A few reports recommended CISD as a viable intervention with school-aged children and adolescents who experienced violence and suicide (e.g., Blackwelder, 1995; O'Hara, Taylor, & Simpson,

1994). Johnson described a school-based approach modeled on four of the original seven CISD phases plus a fifth: introduction, fact-finding, feeling/thought, teaching/educating, and closure phases.

Juhnke (2002) specifically designed the *Adapted Family Debriefing Model* as an assessment and intervention method for elementary, middle, and high school student populations exposed to violence. Under the assumption that parent and student needs often differ, this PD model requires two separate debriefings: one with parents alone; the other with students and parents.

Considering its advantages and disadvantages, it appears that PD should represent only one component within a larger integrated, multi-component crisis management program that covers all phases of disaster. Such a multi-component program consists of the *Critical Incident Stress Management* (CISM; Everly & Mitchell, 1999, 2000). CISM comprises multiple components that functionally span the entire temporal spectrum of a crisis, applied to individuals, small functional groups, families, large groups, organizations, and even communities. The CISM incorporates eight core components: pre-incident preparation, large-scale organizational intervention, defusing, CISD, one-on-one crisis intervention, pastoral crisis intervention, family crisis intervention, and referral and follow-up.

Optimal timing for PD with children is not clear-cut and depends mostly on children's psychological readiness. Some pupils at risk, for example, may not attend available PD activities or pursue a mental health referral early in the disaster recovery process due to denial, delayed onset of symptoms, or a personal perception that their response does not constitute a significant impairment. Therefore, we prefer to incorporate elements of PD at different stages of the intervention. Some of the more educational elements should be incorporated during the primary and early secondary levels of intervention, in the students' briefing, and in the classroom-activated guidance and support. This multi-level approach allows students the choice of active participation according to their extent of neediness, anxiety, and defensiveness. Students whose distress seems to continue may be referred at the next stages by sensitive teachers or their parents for therapeutic group interventions that incorporate psychological debriefing elements, or for additional individual therapy (as outlined in Chapter 14). This more integrative use of psychological debriefing allows more time than a single session for appropriate processing. It also provides a more continuous intimate interpersonal involvement with a caring helper.

When delivered, PD should be closely tailored to children's emotional and cognitive developmental level (Stallard, 2000). For example, children up to about the age of 11 may find it difficult to conceptualize and explore abstract issues and are more concerned with factual information and observable behavior. Preschool and primary grade pupils may have an egocentric magical belief that they are somewhat responsible for what happened. PD with these children may therefore need to focus much more on describing the actual event and correcting any factual misunderstandings. Also, debriefing of professionals must adapt the PD procedure's language to children's comprehension levels (e.g., replacing the term "symptoms" with more concrete examples) and to their difficulty in identifying feelings and sensations. To avoid direct attempts to elicit feelings, which may be deleterious for some children, PD should employ the use of drawings or other indirect expression modes to ventilate feelings and thoughts. Puppets can tell an imaginary story, connected in some subtle way to reality. A distinct phase can be added to specifically encourage the children to think of anything that they did that helped, even slightly (Lahad & Cohen, 1998), to underscore their multidimensional positive coping.

Older children from about the age of 11 are able to handle more abstract concepts and thus may be more aware of issues such as threat to life and survivor guilt. Adolescents may be more concerned with hypothetical and metaphysical issues. Thus, PD with adolescents can include abstract issues that challenge their internal cognitive schemata such as self-blame, survivor guilt, and accountability to allow causal attributions to be reappraised (Casswell, 1997; Stallard, 2000).

In sum, if well planned, delivered by experienced, well-trained practitioners, not mandatory, carefully timed according to recipients' psychological readiness, developmentally adapted, and used as a part of multifaceted crisis intervention plan, PD should be well received by most participants (Bisson, McFarlane, & Rose, 2000; Everly & Mitchell, 2000). A crucial factor in successful application, which is often neglected, comprises the adequate pre-debriefing preparation of the group leader or co-leaders (Dyregrov, 1996).

At the indicated secondary preventive intervention level, within a comprehensive school-based disaster response plan, adequate provisions must be made for readily available treatment and aftercare interventions targeting those children for whom preventive interventions did not preclude onset of a disorder. Students who are later identified as having PTSD symptomatology should be referred to more intensive, group or individual school-based treatment or school-linked clinics. Treatment methods are discussed in Chapter 14.

TERTIARY PREVENTIVE INTERVENTION LEVEL

An additional level of intervention necessary during the recovery phase comprises tertiary prevention. As defined here, school-based tertiary intervention represents the activities applied after victims' acute symptomatology has been eased. These activities aim to minimize residual effects and prevent relapse by stabilizing those who have been hospitalized or have experienced maladjustment and who have received treatment in a protective environment and are now resuming regular activities.

When referred to in this context, tertiary prevention aims mainly at facilitating the academic and social reintegration of these children towards, upon, and after their return to school. This joint cooperative endeavor involves the client in the school (e.g., teachers, peers, administrative staff), the mediator (e.g., psychologist, school counselor, social worker), and the treating professional (e.g., physician, psychiatrist, other clinician). A two-way flow of relevant information and the provision of consultation comprise crucial elements in the child's successful readjustment. These range from sharing information with the absent pupil about the school and class, through helping him or her with the recovery of previously held academic and social skills and competencies, to the acquisition of new skills needed under the circumstances, to the modification of environmental characteristics shown to impede reintegration.

However, tertiary prevention may also refer to a preventive intervention with students who continue to manifest trauma-related psychological difficulties in the long run, or who show a delayed trauma reaction despite the earlier preventive measures (see Chapter 14). These interventions are preventive in counteracting further development of mental health risk.

The main ideas outlined thus far through the 7-level preventive intervention model may be summarized via the intervention flowchart presented in Figure 2. The flowchart may serve as an example of a possible basic response plan for a school disaster. Such a plan should be adapted to the needs and resources of the local school. It should be further developed and readjusted periodically, especially during the anticipatory period and in the postdisaster period to enable proper response to changing needs. Note that the interventions should be viewed as a continuum without clear-cut distinctions in terms of their timeline. Several intervention levels overlap and should be initiated simultaneously, as in the case of the immediate organizational, the primary, and the early secondary preventive interventions.

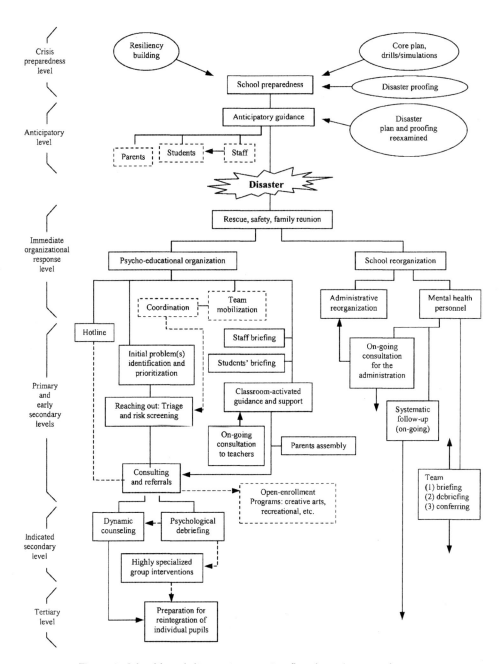

Figure. 2. School-based disaster intervention flowchart: An example.

138

Chapter 12

Active, Positive, and Expressive Activities That Foster Students' Adaptive Coping and Processing

This chapter elaborates on the specifics of a variety of activities enacted by various school personnel during the different stages of dealing with a traumatic event.

STUDENT ACTIVATION ON PROSOCIAL ACTIVITIES

Considering the healing power of giving, schools should first lead students to observe and celebrate others' efforts (e.g., the heroic acts of courageous people following the September 11 attack) and then encourage students to plan and participate in volunteering activities or other tasks that contribute to the class, school, or community. Schools should devise ways to foster prosocial action that suits the situation, location, budget, and student ages. Students can participate in fundraising and donation events such as making and selling home-baked cookies, hand-drawn banners, or teddy bears with personal notes about the disaster victims attached. In certain disasters, like during a flood, children can become actively involved in simple tasks such as becoming messengers and refreshment bringers to the rescue team. When dealing with the death of a classmate or teacher, students can become involved in making a class scrapbook or memorial wall.

Another recommended activity entails encouraging students to create a simple crisis response manual for another school or for a younger age group in the same school. In class, students can review and document people, objects, or resources they feel may have helped them and may help someone else in a similar situation. Classmates become actively involved in discussing candidate resources for inclusion in the manual and in examining the extent to which their needs were met and their recommendations for the future. Allowing students to create something that others can use may promote an active, purposeful, future-oriented outlook and reduce feelings of vulnerability as they transform from "victims" to "experts."

INDIRECT SCHOOL-BASED PSYCHOEDUCATIONAL METHODS

Traumatic events exacerbate excited affects and stimulate powerful projections and fantasies; research findings indicate that survivors encode traumatic experiences in encapsulated nonverbal imagery (Stone, 1998). Although children may be unable to talk about or directly express their overwhelming feelings, they can often address these through indirect expressive and creative forms such as drawing, music, dance, play, and free writing. Nonverbal and non-interpretive school interventions can promote self-recovery. Teachers, teachers of the arts, and volunteering expressive therapists, in consultation with the school's mental health professionals, can help students express emotions, progressively approach traumatic reminders, distance themselves from their feelings by objectifying and containing them in art forms, talk about the images and related feelings, and give some meaning to the confusion of the external environment (Stone, 1998). When used in class or as group projects, the expressive arts open up lines of communication among the students themselves as well as between them and the caring supervising adults (teacher or mental health professional). We will next describe further several of the more common, cost-effective, indirect, semi-structured interventions that schools can employ following a traumatic incident, including expressive writing; humor; expressive arts; graffiti; bibliotherapy, biblioguidance, and storytelling; and nature-assisted activities.

Expressive Writing

As an indirect psychoeducational preventive intervention, expressive writing comprises a non-evaluative process carried out either alone or in a group setting and initiated either by students themselves or by a teacher or counselor. Writing about emotional topics correlates with a reduction in distress because it decreases inhibitory processes, thus constituting a coping strategy that effectively addresses the need for disclosure. Although affect disclosure comprises a powerful therapeutic agent that may account for some percentage of the variance in the healing process, writing goes much beyond the mere expression of pent-up emotions to an inclusion of the role of thoughts and insight (Niederhoffer & Pennebaker,

2002) without sharing it. Writing about the thoughts and feelings surrounding a trauma may bring about a change in cognitive processes by "translating" the experience into language during the writing (Pennebaker, 1997). Cognitive-behavioral paradigms suggest that expressive writing facilitates cognitive processing of traumatic memory, which leads to affective and behavioral change (Pennebaker, Colder, & Sharp, 1990). Research with children suggests that free writing consists of a practical, cost-effective procedure to use with schools in war zones and may be readily incorporated into the school curriculum (Klingman, 1985a, 1985b). Classroom writing assignments can also serve as "quiet time," enabling the teacher to talk individually with students who need more individual reassurance.

In the school setting, expressive writing allows students the privacy and freedom to express themselves without concern for others' reactions. Students can decide whether or not to share their writing, with whom, when, and where. Nevertheless, classroom writing often becomes a shared group experience and may even be published in a school newspaper. When communicated to a group of others sharing similar concerns, writing provides a standard of normalcy against which students can compare themselves.

A survey of 6- to 11-year-olds' creative products conducted by the Sesame Workshop (creators of educational television programming) after the September 11 attack revealed coping mechanisms in children's writing that had not appeared in predisaster surveys. For example, some children imagined themselves as heroes, writing that they wanted to be able to fly "to stop the bad guys" or "touch a cloud so if someone is about to be hurt I could lift them" [http://www.coping.org/911/pixmood/content.htlm]. In this respect, free writing provides students with a self-help alternative.

Journalistic writing, although not necessarily related to emotional expression, also helps children feel in control of their environment. Reporting and documenting the events and their aftermath in a school newspaper, or constructing a memorial scrapbook for a close victim of disaster, allows children the opportunity to be active and task oriented, creatively express their feelings about the loss, and start the process of closure. Teachers or counselors may also ask survivors to keep a diary about their thoughts, feelings, observations, behaviors, and coping. This medium may be especially helpful when school is temporarily closed and can also later be professionally shared with a professional with the student's/parent's permission in cases of concern.

Writing is not, however, always beneficial (Wright & Chung, 2001). Psychological pain resulting from writing about a traumatic experience may be intolerable for some children. Other issues relate to children's academic skills and difficulties. Students may be frustrated with attempts to express themselves in writing if they do not possess a high degree of verbal ability. Others may avoid writing because of past negative experience with written school assignments or due to learning disabilities such as a disorder of written expression (*DSM-IV*; American Psychiatric Association,

1994). Thus, writing about traumatic experience should not be mandatory but rather suggested and encouraged only as matter of choice for the students. Also, any classroom activity involving writing and drawing about the event must allow time for addressing the associated anxieties involved, otherwise it may further sensitize some of the students rather than habituate them.

Humor

Humorous writing constitutes a valuable expressive tool for some youngsters. Students often utilize humor to reduce stress. Humor has received theoretical endorsement as an adaptive emotion-focused coping technique. Lefcourt and his colleagues (Lefcourt, 2000; Lefcourt & Thomas, 1998) found that humor alters the emotional consequences of stressful events and correlates positively with optimism and positive reframing. Joking about surrounding dangers allows a cathartic expression of stress without directly revealing specific fears (Berk, 1998). Children who use humor to cope can detach themselves from negative emotions. Humor generation, production, and appreciation can provide the emotional distance necessary to gain perspective on a situation. For example, during an extremely tense period of terrorist attacks during the Palestinian uprising in Israel, we witnessed Jerusalem adolescents who incorporated morbid humor and cynicism referring to real dangers into their daily lives. Youngsters related to party invitations with word games reflecting the times: "It's going to be an explosive party." They also would respond to the routine send-off "See you later" with retorts such as "Don't be so sure" or "You never know."

In the class setting, students should be allowed to create caricatures or write humorously about aspects of the traumatic event, and to publish these in the class or school newspaper. It may be important to elaborate on the value of humor in teachers' meetings, and to suggest how (and if) teachers may respond to students' humorous products that adults might find in bad taste.

Expressive Arts

Although well-controlled empirical research has not yet established the therapeutic effect of creative art intervention, expressive arts are widely used, especially the plastic arts, with children in the aftermath of traumatic events. The arts clearly involve generic recovery processes that overlap with many established trauma-related interventions, such as relaxation, gradual exposure, desensitization, cognitive processing and reframing, narrative techniques, and distraction (Johnson, 2000). Many creative art methods comprise child-centered, developmentally appropriate activities that lend themselves to adaptation during the initial recovery period. For example, free work with modeling clay constitutes a stress-free and often stress-relieving activity that does not require verbal discussion of the disaster; children can talk when they reach their own level of comfort and security. Even debris or rubble brought to the classroom can undergo transformation into a unique, lively painted canvas, promoting feelings of doing something "hands-on" and meaningful toward recovery. Another expressive art intervention comprised the decoration of the gas mask boxes by Israeli children during the anticipatory period of the 1991 Gulf War, when they had to carry the kits to school every day for weeks. Decorating the gas mask boxes became a popular class and school project that not only helped disguise the frightening contents and render the boxes less threatening and more personal, but also entailed an artistic project that introduced self-expression and fun into a very tense, anxiety laden, period.

The incorporation of expressive art into posttrauma school-based preventive intervention offers a number of advantages. The art product provides *a sense of distance* from the emotional turmoil, enabling students to deal with the frightening or overly painful issue at hand more easily because the art has brought it out into the open. Children experience *immediate healing effects,* permitting an earlier onset for processing the trauma. Considering the need for a multidimensional approach due to the magnitude and multidimensionality of trauma, art's expressive medium aptly engages *affective, cognitive, and perceptual capacities.* When utilized as a *doing and sharing* process, expressive arts promote feelings of common bonds and normalization. The *flexibility and versatility* of art allow diverse media to be used with individuals, groups, an entire classroom, or a family unit. In group art sessions, caregivers can allow children to funnel their individual as well as their common fears and anxieties into creative expression and work them through. The artwork can be created *inside and/or outside of the classroom,* thus enabling the product to serve as an expressive modality anywhere (e.g., at home), anytime. The finished product can trigger parent-child communication and mutual understanding, forming a *triangular relationship* between the student, parent, and artwork. For some children, especially younger ones, a drawing is "worth a thousand words," expressing fear, confusion, and sorrow that they cannot verbalize, even though they may not really understand all that has happened. In cases where art projects are submitted for exhibition, this promotes a *future-oriented outlook.*

Examples of artwork following the September 11 attack can illustrate its benefits. Children sent their artwork to the Pentagon and to rescue stations (fire, police, paramedic), where recipients gratefully displayed the art in the hallways. Many children's drawings around the U.S. could be seen in school corridors. In Manhattan, while the Stuyvesant High School adjacent to the WTC was closed, its students gathered in Greenwich Village to collectively paint two giant (12-by-80-foot) murals commemorating the tragedy. In addition to appreciating the mural as artwork, many students said that they enjoyed how students of all grades and circles cooperated in the face of adversity (*The Spectator: The Stuyvesant High School Newspaper*, New York, October 2, 2001). The mural painting embodied positive psychology (Seligman, 2002), in that these students reached out to one another and partook in a collective event that moved the students from passivity to active, constructive involvement.

The Sesame Workshop's survey of drawings among children aged 6 to 11 revealed dramatically different pictures in the weeks following the September 11 attack, compared to predisaster pictures. The postdisaster drawings depicted collapsed buildings, fallen planes, soldiers in camouflage, firefighters and police officers, family graveyards, nuclear explosions, and darkness. One child attached a photograph (older children were provided with disposable cameras) of utter blackness to her composition, with the caption "This is a picture of nothing, because the president said we might have a nuclear war and the world will look like this" [http://www.coping.org/911/healing/kidart.htlm].

Not all students feel comfortable drawing, but some other art forms may appeal to them. For example, some children may enjoy creating a collage about the event from magazine or newspaper clippings, including the cut-and-paste activity and discussion around the table about the collage topics (for an illustration of schoolchildren's collage works following trauma, see Klingman et al., 1987). Others may benefit from photographing subjects related to the situation and the recovery process and from creating a photo album for the class or a photography exhibit in the school.

Graffiti

As a creative means of youthful coping with macro-level collective disaster – the assassination of Prime Minister Rabin in Israel in 1995 – Klingman and colleagues (Klingman & Shalev, 2001; Klingman, Shalev et al., 2000) evaluated and discussed graffiti. The examination of conventional and unconventional symbols as well as texts revealed, overall, that graffiti represented spontaneous and authentic feelings of loss and "spontaneous memorialization." Graffiti can also comprise a preplanned project within the school setting, presented as a wall composition or memorial wall. Such graffiti activity encompasses, beyond artistic expression, a natural support system (the school), social support (peers, teachers), communality, continuity (the educational framework), expectancy, and spontaneous healing processes promoted through creativity.

Bibliotherapy, Biblioguidance, and Storytelling

Bibliotherapy involves directed reading and discussion of carefully chosen texts related, directly or indirectly, to the current situation, concerns, and problems. Relating to characters and situations in the text, students can confront deeper messages beyond the plot and, from an emotional distance, apply lessons learned from the texts to their own experience and difficulties. Bibliotherapy especially suits children who have difficulty verbalizing their thoughts and feelings. Kubovi (1982) presented the application of bibliotherapy during war and its aftermath. Offered within the supportive classroom setting as a *collaborative process* between the teacher and the group, therapeutic bibliotherapy may serve as a middle course between uncontrolled or unstructured ventilation of feelings and defensive, denial-like, avoidance of disturbing, traumatic elements of the event. This technique involves the student's identification with a story character, projection of feelings and thoughts onto that character, and experiencing psychological relief, self-reflection, and insight. The classroom discussion creates awareness that others have similar feelings and thoughts. When uncontrolled or difficult-to-handle emotional ventilation predominates, the teacher or school counselor redirects students to the text's contents (e.g., the story characters), thereby allowing intellectualization, interposing a requisite distance from upsetting issues. The students may then be directed to focus on coping strategies (e.g., help-seeking behaviors, problem-solving techniques) and solutions to problems, as well as new values and attitudes leading to trauma growth. Bibliotherapy also enables teachers and counselors to feel "safe" in approaching sensitive issues in a classroom context and to control their own emotional reactions in the classroom, by returning to the familiar text when necessary. Text selection should consider the story or poem's relevance to the current situation, the students' reading level, and the students' ability to identify with the plot, setting, dialogue, and characters in view of their emotional and chronological age. The text should also reflect positive, age-appropriate coping strategies and an optimistic, surmountable presentation of the traumatic event (Jalongo, 1983; Pardeck & Pardeck, 1984; Rubin, 1978).

Biblioguidance comprises a similar medium (Klingman, 1992b, 1993), but differs from bibliotherapy in that its main purpose consists of providing information. Various kinds of information can be· conveyed through assigned and shared reading. For example, a specially designed story-and-coloring booklet helped explain chemical warfare terms and gas mask protection procedures to Israeli youngsters during the 1991 Gulf War (Klingman, 1992). Similarly, FEMA provides an updated bibliography of books on disaster for children according to age level and language (http://www.fema.gov/kids/teacher.htm). Disaster relief workbooks can also be downloaded from the Internet (http://www.cphc-sf.org/disaster_books.htm).

Another related intervention method for young or nonverbal children comprises *storytelling*. Students receive encouragement to tell their own story of the traumatic event using a wide variety of media, in the presence of significant supportive others such as teachers. Storytelling can be aloud, via drawings or printed pictures, in coloring books, through dramatization of "radio play" (e.g., pretending to be a radio announcer), with hand pup-

pets, or using toys. Telling about feelings helps the child validate and normalize emotions, which contributes to desensitization and effectively de-
stigmatizes the child (Kupersmidt, Shahinfar, & Voegler-Lee, 2002). At the
end of group telling of a trauma-related story, children can be asked to
invent an ending to the story; the class context is conducive to sharing and
discussion of the various endings. Children can draw a "class storybook,"
illustrating the disaster, and arrive together at decisions about contents.
Older students can prepare books individually.

Nature-Assisted Intervention Activities

We have elaborated in Chapter 8 on the idea that the process of coping
with a traumatic event presents children and adults with an opportunity
for psychological growth. This growth may be enhanced by activities that
involve the children in new explorations and appreciation of their physical
environment and in the development of awareness to their own potential
contributions to the quality of life.

Borrowing from a nature therapy approach (Nebbe, 2000), numerous
school-based nature-assisted activities can be devised for trauma-related
preventive recovery interventions. This educational activity should be
planned together with nature experts (possibly as part of school environmental education programs) and delivered by educational staff, but should
be therapeutically goal directed and supervised by a mental health professional. Its therapeutic value lies in promoting active coping, creativity,
caring, and a future-oriented outlook. Gardening activities such as potting,
caring for, and protecting plants may increase students' mobility by granting them more freedom in an outdoor environment. Gentle, successful car-
etaking of animals or plants may enhance students' sense of control,
responsibility, confidence, and self-worth. Nature-related knowledge
acquisition and skill development can enhance children's self-esteem. Students may follow the self-recovery of a plant, thus cognitively and experi-
entially learning about trauma and trauma-induced growth. Helping a
plant grow or a domestic animal survive can give an individual purpose;
this and other nature-related experiences may provide some children with
life-renewing energy. Watching and enjoying nature, whether puppies
playing or flowers blooming, can be stimulating, fun, and relaxing; as is
watching an aquarium full of fish (Beck & Katcher, 1983); and even viewing a natural environment on video or still photographs (Ulrich, 1993).

One nature-assisted intervention in the war-torn former Yugoslavia
organized students in a garden-planting club. Flower planting involved
talking about an expectation that the students would be around to see and
nurture the blooms. Activities included finding ways to protect their plants
from theft or destruction during an enemy attack; students then could
apply some of the same skills to protect themselves (Berk, 1998).

Another example constitutes a combined botany and art project initiated in Israel for bereaved immigrant families whose lives were shattered by the sudden loss of a family member. This model can be adjusted to school-based intervention (Pardess, 2002a). Students in this project learned about processes of regeneration and rebuilding following a forest fire or other natural trauma. A nature hike for first-hand observation intended to evoke responses and facilitate a discussion about survival. Contents included how difficult it was for these plants and trees to go on living, their capacity to heal themselves, and healing processes that are often hidden from view. The intervention facilitator used a tree as a metaphor to relate non-intrusively to the traumatic experience. The metaphor allowed distancing and buffered the potentially re-sensitizing impact of direct confrontation and disclosure of painful emotions. Following the nature hike, students participated in an art session involving the drawing of trees, entitled "Telling the story of the hurt tree." This approach currently plays an integral part in the Israel Crisis Management Center's posttrauma growth activity program for bereaved victims in the aftermath of terrorist attacks (Pardess, 2002b). The center conducts multi-sensual nature hikes combined with discussion group sessions led by an expert botanist, focusing on regeneration and rebuilding following a nature trauma. This is followed by a "testimonial" art activity, in which children draw and tell the story of the recovering tree, thus acknowledging their loss and constructing a personal narrative that may be shared with others.

Science Projects

Recreating a natural disaster (tornado, flood) in the laboratory offers an appropriate science activity that can help children understand why and how disaster occurred. This is especially desired when children feel anxious about a repeat of the incident or feel a loss of trust in others. Strategic games may help achieve a sense of intellectual control in regard to deliberate human disasters. For example, an experiment carried out with Israeli elementary school students following a terrorist attack (Ophir, 1980) found that the ad hoc creation of a simulation board game significantly reduced students' state anxiety. Students took an active part in creating and structuring the game, which included moving security and terrorist forces around the board. Via role taking, they learned the best positions for the security forces in and around town, weighed different security measures taken by citizens and by children in particular, and assessed the probability of terrorists reaching the game's neighborhood, school, class, and homes. Such actions enabled students to positively focus some of their energy on planning, taking action, and gaining a sense of control.

SPIRITUALITY AND RELIGION AS COPING RESOURCES

Spiritual and religious coping comprise another active resource that can be tapped in attempting to support the recovery of school personnel, the student body, and parents. Trauma can cause a person to reexamine long-held values and basic beliefs that give meaning to life as well as to reexamine dilemmas, predicaments, and life issues in light of the current disaster. Coping with shattered assumptions involves a confrontational strategy of finding meaning in one's postdisaster world (see personality factors impacting children's psychological responses to disaster in Chapter 3).

In our experiences with traumatic events, we have observed both religious faith and philosophical perspectives becoming resources that play an important role in coping with trauma. People the world over often visit places of worship more frequently after a traumatic event even in secular societies. For many families and school staff, crisis can be made more manageable by reliance on religious beliefs. Studies reveal a generally positive correlation between religion and mental and physical health, suggesting that religion may play a helpful role in the coping process, offering benefits even beyond those obtained through non-religious coping methods (Pargament et al., 1999).

Considering that in some countries the division of church and state is strictly observed, religious schools may benefit more than public schools from religious coping resources. Adoption of a crisis-sensitive curriculum in religious schools (Roberts, 2001) allows students opportunities to discuss crises, debate crisis-related problems, and explore alternatives in relation to faith.

Nevertheless, students may find that nondenominational religious practices give meaning to the event and provide a sense of secure attachment, control, or optimism. Ad hoc school-based voluntary gatherings may comprise non-religious assemblies or nondenominational religious services for which specific prayers may be selected or original prayers may be composed. The avenue of prayer may be especially welcome when children's natural support systems are temporarily helpless or absent. On the other hand, prayer can be intrusive and ill-advised when ill timed (Woodruff, 2002). Something as innocent as asking students to pray for a disaster victim who subsequently died may increase a sensitive student's emotional proximity to the event and may lead to a sense of culpability if the prayers "fail" (Nader & Muni, 2002).

Many people who reject formal religion as such nonetheless consider themselves to be spiritual human beings. Spirituality is a term used to refer to religious attitudes and practices as well as non-religious experiential dimensions. From a non-religious frame of reference, spirituality encompasses a "philosophical" self-examination and "a search for wisdom" (Lahav, 1996). In this sense, a crisis can cause non-religious individuals to reexamine their values and the basic beliefs that heretofore gave meaning to life. Applying spiritual values and resources in the management of a traumatic experience, employing faith-based guidance, and implementing pastoral crisis intervention in disasters have recently gained acceptance among interventionists (e.g., Everly, 2000a, 2000b). Schools may wish to carefully consider the role of spirituality in their search for means to foster students' active coping and processing of disaster.

SUMMARY

It is impossible to present in this one chapter the full range of school-based, teacher-led educational and psychoeducational interventions. Furthermore, different types of disaster necessitate different, often unexpected types of interventions and tools. Beyond well-established strategies, familiar tools, and learned techniques as partially described in this chapter, it is essential to rely on the teaching staff's creativity. Teachers as instructors and educators already possess the ability to reach out to students and often wield a powerfully protective and preventative effect on them. Every effort should be made to mobilize all school-based resources and encourage staff creativity to help children adaptively cope with the ravages of mass disaster. In this regard, it should be stressed that the appropriate role for the mental health professional lies in indirect bolstering of the school system and school staff rather than displacing them.

Chapter 13

School-Based Preventive Interventions with Parents Around Mass Trauma

In Chapter 7, we have delineated the central role that parents play in the child's process of coping with traumatic events. Parents' ability to buffer the trauma's impact, and their possible unintentional contribution to the exacerbation of the child''s maladaptive reactions, necessitate parental inclusion in preventive intervention whenever possible. Parental inclusion may take the form of enlisting them as significant partners in efforts to facilitate children's coping and processing of trauma, while concomitantly addressing the parents' own trauma-related needs. Although such inclusion is well supported by the literature and acknowledged by most trauma experts, many school-based intervention programs continue to neglect the parental component (Chemtob, Nakashima & Carlson, 2002; March, Amaya-Jackson, Murray and Schulte, 1998).

The active, multifaceted roles that parents can play in their children's recovery may run the gamut, including: (a) offering emotional support and soothing; (b) organizing a stable, regulating environment; (c) opening channels of communication and using empathic listening to the child's account and reactions to the traumatic event; (d) helping the child make sense out of the experience by correcting misperceptions, exploring meaning, and offering new perspectives regarding the unusual events; (e) relaying optimism and resourcefulness; (f) exploring, discovering, and prompting family members' strengths; (g) increasing family cohesiveness; (h) detecting signs of traumatic stress in their children and helping to alleviate the distressing symptoms; and (i) seeking help for long-term unremitting posttraumatic symptoms and acting as co-therapists.

Schools comprise natural partners in some of these tasks and offer potential resources in guiding and supporting parents during the intervention process. Parents' feelings of connection to the school and their trust in its personnel may be considered important sources for their own coping ability as parents. In this chapter, we elaborate on the specific plans and interventions that may facilitate the partnership between parents and schools around trauma, and that may best support parents in their challenging role of supporting their children in recovering from trauma. These include establishing parent-school collaboration; issues related to parent-child reunification after a disaster; the delivery of communication, crisis intervention, and consultation services for parents; and the implementation of group interventions for parents.

BUILDING COLLABORATION BETWEEN
PARENTS AND SCHOOLS

An ongoing partnership between parents and school personnel in regular times constitutes an important prerequisite for smooth collaboration in times of crisis. Collaboration is crucial during crisis to improve children's physical and psychological safety and the well being of the adults themselves. At times of disaster and trauma, schools must consider the central role of the ecological approach, which espouses coordination between school personnel and parents, in understanding and meeting children's mental health needs (Benedeck, 1979; Norris et al., 2002b). A genuine parent-school partnership is based on the school's acknowledgement of parents' central role in the child's development and on the school's respect for parents as sharing complementary educational roles with the school personnel. In such a partnership, the school updates parents on ongoing activities, issues, and plans; encourages mutual problem solving procedures; and welcomes parents' input, contributions, and even criticisms concerning particular issues relating to their children. The parents, in turn, respect and value the contribution of the school, and become involved in cooperative efforts to promote their mutual goals. Well-established attitudes of acknowledgment, acceptance, and respect toward parents' important roles will lead naturally to the school's inclusion of parents in the preparedness phase of devising strategic plans to deal with various disasters. Crisis intervention specialists (Brock et al., 2001; Pitcher & Poland, 1992) seem to agree that crisis teams and school officials should work proactively with parents prior to and during crisis rather than waiting for parents' advances and initiatives. A proactive stance advocates the inclusion of parent representatives as an integral part in the school's crisis team at its planning stage. Additionally, parent volunteers for special emergency roles and tasks may also be designated ahead of time, based on the parents' professional capabilities or their availability and proximity to the school. For example, while preparing in Israel for a possible war between the USA and Iraq in the winter of 2003, parents who worked in the physical proximity of schools agreed to serve as volunteers to help younger children don gas masks in emergency cases of suspected chemical attack. Furthermore, school policy around major emergency issues needs to be on record and discussed with parents, such as school safety; procedures for school evacuation, closure, or displacement; pre-established means of communication with parents; emergency handling of casualties; and ways to psychologically process trauma. This is based both on the parents' right to know and on the need for parents to be psychologically ready and logistically cooperative in times of crisis.

The school system may gain additional support from the parent body by providing opportunities for parents to volunteer in a variety of roles and activities relevant not only to the anticipatory or immediate organizational response, but also to the different levels of intervention in the aftermath of trauma. Parents can, for example, actively take part in contacting families of children who have not returned to school when it reopened, or they may participate according to their talents in psychoeducational activities initiated to process the traumatic experience, such as expressive arts projects. This sort of collaboration empowers the parents and creates a special bond between parents, teachers, and students.

COORDINATION AND ORGANIZATION OF REUNIFICATION BETWEEN PARENTS AND CHILDREN

Reuniting students with their families as soon as possible during the immediate postimpact phase is in most crisis situations a recommended intervention and primary prevention practice. This is based on previously reviewed literature (see Chapter 7) highlighting the protective effects of the family cohesiveness on the adjustment of children exposed to traumatic events. Younger children's reunion with their parents should be a priority. The first sight of a parent may cause relief or may increase stress; for example, children have often described an escalation of fear or anxiety in response to seeing the extremely distressed look on a parent's face (Pynoos & Nader, 1989). Therefore, prior to the reunion, parents may benefit from a very brief transition period in which the crisis team can assist parents to compose themselves before they join their children (Nader & Pynoos, 1993).

The process of reuniting with parents needs to be planned and monitored so that the release of children is carried out in as orderly and calm a fashion as possible under the given circumstances. The process needs to be supervised (schools should release the children only to individuals previously identified as authorized to pick them up) and clearly documented (release forms need to be prepared in advance and be readily available). Previously planned crowd control and traffic management for the schoolyard and parking area need to be instituted and readjusted according to the particular circumstances. Another important preparation by school staff members comprises prearrangement with caregivers for the staff's own personal children at home, for the duration of time that staff members may be retained in school due to the crisis situation.

COMMUNICATION, CRISIS INTERVENTION, AND CONSULTATION SERVICES FOR PARENTS

A well-prepared school crisis team should plan various communication modes for implementation in the aftermath of a disaster, and should establish an infrastructure to underlie the expected calls and referrals from the student body and their families. Immediate needs for crisis intervention with parents may include traditional consultation and nontraditional roles for the school mental health professionals at the family and the group level.

Planning Communication Modes

During the immediate post-impact phase when a disaster involves school-children, the school crisis team must address parents' urgent needs for updated information and guidelines for action, as well as parents' additional needs for support and education. Communication is the key. In the wake of a disaster, the school must disseminate clear and timely information to parents about the available channels of communication with the school. Such channels may involve an initial parent assembly to give updates on facts, casualties, and plans for the coming minutes and hours. Other channels include telephone and written communication with parents, school websites, telephone hotlines, and even the use of local mass media. The communication of immediate updated information about the traumatic event can prevent rumors, confusion, and incubation of anxiety. Knowledge of facts and reassurance can help calm parents, so that they can collaborate in the initial postdisaster interventions, first focusing on students' physical safety and then on soothing and psychologically stabilizing their children. Clear communication may prevent "interfering" behaviors by well-meaning but ill-informed and anxious parents, who may withdraw their children from school, based on rumors of an anticipated disaster, or may even undermine rescue and recovery efforts at a time of disaster. In line with the generic principle of continuity (see Chapter 9), after the establishment of physical safety, school communications should clearly state the crucial importance of preserving and restoring routines as soon as possible. Later, the school will need to issue updates regarding the return to school activities, safety issues, logistical and psychoeducational information (e.g., on funeral attendance, special parent meetings). Clarification and coordination of immediate and future plans and needed actions may further help parents regain a sense of control. At times, communication channels will develop and change over an extended period of time, as different requirements emerge and as the school consolidates its plans for dealing with the traumatic events.

Immediate Crisis Intervention and Consultation

During the impact and the immediate postdisaster phases, some families will need immediate help. Parents and especially mothers seem to be frequent users of telephone hotlines and media counseling programs, especially during times of war involving unfamiliar threats (Raviv, 1993). The well-timed availability of phone consultation or an urgent appointment with a mental health professional from the school's team (i.e., the school counselor or school psychologist), or from an affiliated agency, may help parents prevent many situations from getting out of hand. Direct simple advice and a soothing perspective can help confused parents organize their behavior.

For example, for the period immediately following a terrorist incident that killed three children who attended one Jerusalem school, the school's mental health team, aided by two collaborating professional volunteers, made themselves available to parents' phone calls after school hours. On the day of the victims' funerals, the father of one adolescent student called the volunteering professional late at night. He was extremely concerned because his daughter was crying, seemed upset, and was having difficulties falling asleep. He was debating whether to take her to the hospital emergency room, or to go out and buy non-prescription sleeping pills. Following some clarification of the girl's situation, it appeared that the father was overreacting out of anxiety. A normalizing explanation regarding the girl's distress and insomnia helped the father understand his daughter's need to process her many thoughts and feelings. Rather than recommending medication, the professional suggested that the father sit by her bedside and offer to listen to her or calm her for as long as necessary that night. He was asked to call back in the morning. Upon doing so, he reported that his communicating to his daughter his willingness to sit by her bed even for the whole night had a dramatic relaxing effect on her. She fell asleep shortly afterwards.

Another example comprises ongoing communication with parents regarding children's participation in schoolmates' funerals. After consulting with its mental health team, the school should communicate (in writing or via a group meeting, and in special cases by personal phone calls from the teachers) its recommendations for funeral attendance to the parents (see Chapter 9), while obtaining input from each family regarding individual children's participation. Inasmuch as the usefulness of children's participation in such rituals may depend, beyond the child's age and closeness to the victim, on the support of available significant adults, the school may ask parents to accompany their child through the funeral experience and may offer to prepare parents for this role.

Nontraditional Crisis Activities with Parents

At times, the nature of an emergency requires that school mental health professionals become an active part of the emergency service personnel and be involved in social, physical, logistical, and organizational activities that differ from their traditional therapeutic roles. For example, school psychologists may find themselves waiting with parents immediately after the news of a disaster has surfaced, when specific information regarding casualties remains unclear. This occurred in a number of well-publicized incidents in Israel that involved fatal accidents or terrorist shootings among different groups of children while on school outings. Similarly, during a 1995 wildfire in the Judea Hill forest that led to the evacuation of many homes and villages, school psychologists were present at the evacuation center, helping to soothe and emotionally support evacuated families. The psychologists also helped tend to various pressing physical and organizational needs such as food, medications, diapers, and supervision of children. Only later did they resume their role of organizing mental health services for high-risk families, and consultation to the educational system. Likewise, after the 1991 Oakland Hills firestorm in the USA, mental health professionals accompanied families to view the damage to their homes, while providing support and comfort during the process (Gordon et al., 1999). Similarly, in the wake of Hurricane Andrew in Florida in 1992, the mental health staff discerned parental stress among the relocated disaster victims and therefore helped set up child care provisions in the emergency centers, to provide diversion for the children and free parents to deal with the many challenging tasks they faced (Gordon et al., 1999).

In Israel school psychologists were occasionally enlisted after a terrorist bus explosion to support family members in their search for the fate of their loved ones, including a visit to the morgue. These psychologists used their experience in crisis intervention and in working with various school populations to adapt themselves to the changing needs of different individuals at moments of extreme stress and crisis. They managed to offer their empathy and supportive presence, legitimized people's reactions, and stayed close by until communication was established with other family members.

Group Interventions

At a somewhat later stage, usually when the school is ready to move from the immediate organizational response level to the level of primary preventive interventions, related to the recovery phase, the school will need to organize both large-group and small-group parent guidance meetings, as elaborated later in this chapter. Large-group meetings allow the school to share information regarding the traumatic event and regarding planned actions to help children cope with its aftermath. Such large-group meetings often provide an opportunity to educate parents about their children's psychological reactions and needs. These meetings also allow parents an opportunity to ask questions, exchange ideas, and voice their needs and concerns. The small-group format, which lends itself to more personal and bi-directional communication as part of the processing of trauma, better suits the needs of parents who were more directly affected by the traumatic event. The small counseling groups provide a more intimate context for emotional sharing, support, empowerment, and specific problem solving. Multifamily groups are another, less frequently used option. We will next provide some specific guidelines for suggested contents and structure of these intervention formats, focusing in more detail on the most common types of group intervention: large parent groups and small parent groups.

LARGE-GROUP INTERVENTION WITH PARENTS SUBSEQUENT TO A DISASTER

Following a disaster or traumatic event, parent assemblies fulfill several important functions: as a forum for communication between the school administration and parents; as a peer support forum for communication and sharing among the parents themselves; and as an optimal setting for parental education and guidance. In line with the generic principle of immediacy, assemblies should be held within a few days of the event, after the school has achieved initial stabilization and reorganization. Depending on the circles of vulnerability identified for a particular traumatic incident (see Figure 1, in Chapter 11), the invited parents may be those of a specific grade level, of several grade levels, or of the entire student body, in line with the generic principle of sense of community.

The large-group forum affords an important primary preventive intervention. It offers school officials an opportunity to delineate logistical and practical procedures, psychoeducational measures, and social activities to parents, including:

Organizational measures:

1. Communicating the school staff's sense of confidence and control over situational demands (in line with the generic principle of expectancy).
2. Providing accurate and updated details of the event and its impact, so as to dispel possible rumors and to disseminate accurate information.
3. Indicating the steps already taken by the school and the mental health team to cope with the event, and additional planned actions.

4. Clarifying the challenges facing the school in the present and in the near future.

Psychoeducational measures:

5. Emphasizing the staff's interest in parents' concerns and needs.
6. Making suggestions for complementary at home and at school measures in regard to the children (such as application of the continuity principle, efforts to engage the children in helping activities or to strengthen their social peer network.)
7. Offering lectures and small-group follow-up regarding issues of common concern to parents (the impact of the traumatic experience on children; how to respond to children's reactions, concerns, and new behaviors, etc.).
8. Circulating a needs assessment questionnaire to be completed by parents at the assembly, to tap the more quiet parents' needs and to receive input into the planning of services for children and parents.

Social measures:

9. Extending an invitation to parents to become active volunteers in addressing the school community's needs.

We will elaborate next on some of the parent assembly's psychoeducational and social functions.

Airing and Addressing Parents' Concerns

A major function of the parent assembly comprises the opportunity for the school administration to encourage parents to raise questions and share their general concerns regarding the school's functioning and its ability to ensure the children's welfare. Some of these concerns may be addressed immediately by providing relevant information, whereas other concerns require further discussion to delineate an appropriate mechanism for addressing them. For example, the assembly may set in motion the appointment of a special parent committee to check safety issues, or may empower the PTA to take a specific stance vis-à-vis the local board of education.

Additional concerns about parents' own functioning and their children's adjustment may also be shared. Verbal expression of such concerns at the meeting may help the crisis team to plan models for immediate psychological support for parents. The distribution of a needs assessment questionnaire offers a structured written alternative that particularly targets those parents who do not actively participate in the assembly. Cohen (2000) found that parents of junior high school students welcomed responding to such questionnaires prior to a parent assembly that was held 10 days after a terrorist bomb explosion killed three of the school's students. The parents willingly described their children's coping and their own concerns, and they even asked to be identified by name, although they were initially asked to complete the questionnaires anonymously. Parents also reported that the questionnaire itself served as a catalyst for initiating conversations with their adolescents regarding the traumatic event.

Educating Parents in Coping with Disaster and Trauma

Many parents feel that they lack the knowledge and skills necessary to help their children in times of crisis and can benefit from direct psychoeducation concerning the management of their child's posttraumatic symptoms (AACAP, 1998; Cohen, Berliner & March, 2000). Although printed materials and websites may provide parents with general relevant information regarding children's coping with trauma, the experience of being together with other parents in a school setting for educative purposes appears to hold added benefits. A group setting furnishes psychological and social support via the sharing and ventilation of feelings and via the experience of such feelings as universal. Additionally, sharing and receiving information with other parents about the children's reactions may help parents gain a new perspective on the situation; such as finding relief in learning how the children support each other, and how common some of the stress reactions are. A group setting may also be conducive to learning new skills through exposure to the reports of interventions undertaken by various parents, as well as for individual and group problem solving and empowerment.

During a parent assembly, a lecture by an experienced mental health professional (preferably a member of the school's crisis team) can optimally deliver the knowledge base relevant to coping with trauma to a large group of affected parents. Nevertheless, the large gathering should break up afterwards into small groups for the more intimate processing of feelings and concerns, and for the assimilation of the presented ideas and principles. The mere ability to talk about the trauma may promote a reduction in parental avoidance tendencies, and may foster parents' psychological readiness to deal with their children's avoidance.

Generally, the large-group lecture should address the knowledge base relevant to central issues that concern all invited parents. These issues usually include an understanding of the impact of the traumatic experience on children; the meaning of children's behavioral changes; how to respond to children's reactions, concerns, and new behaviors; and how to foster children's adaptive coping. The major messages to be delivered to parents encompass normalization, the typical course of recovery, explanations for stress responses, the importance of acknowledging and reinforcing the child's strengths, the importance of the recovery environment, the need to continue monitoring the child's long- term adjustment, and information regarding resources.

Normalization

The lecturer must first and foremost emphasize a message of normalization, emphasizing that children's patterns of reaction to abnormal situations that overwhelm their habitual coping systems will characteristically include a wide range of atypical behaviors. Typical behavioral changes include school avoidance, clinging, separation anxiety, fears, sleeping problems, concentration difficulties, irritability or jumpiness, misbehavior at school or home, physical complaints, feelings of sadness, and not wanting to play with friends (NIMH, 2000). The message of legitimization can crucially lessen parental anxiety, which in itself may exacerbate children's sense of insecurity.

A frequently asked question in parent groups relates to evaluating children's progress in processing the trauma. Some parents worry because their child does not exhibit any apparent reactions to the traumatic event, and shows no indications of processing the trauma, whereas others worry because the child seems extremely preoccupied by the event, to the exclusion of many everyday activities (Cohen, 2000). The lecturer may guide parents to expect movements between a reflective mode and a coping mode and to consider professional consultation only when the child demonstrates persistent and rigid avoidance of either returning to normal coping or facing trauma-related materials and cues. Parents may also be directed to observe and monitor even slight signs of their child's attempts to rework trauma memories and reactions, as well as advances in resuming more ordinary functioning (see description of parent training in child observation skills below).

Typical Course of Recovery

To increase tolerance of current symptoms and to enhance optimism, the lecturer should communicate expectations for a gradual reduction in children's symptoms, as well as expected variability in individual timelines. Symptoms may be presented as useful mechanisms for eliciting help, for strengthening relationships, and for self-discovery. Emphasis should be placed on long- term processes of coping with the adverse experience, and on increasing resilience, benefit finding, and trauma-induced growth, as outlined in Chapter 8.

Explanations for Stress Responses

The lecturer can utilize various theoretical approaches to help parents understand different aspects of children's stress responses to trauma. Psychobiologically-based explanations may clarify some posttraumatic phenomena as manifestations of the body's attempt to fight, flee, or freeze. The realization that traumatized people may, at least for a while, experience life as a continuation of the trauma, and remain in a state of constant alert for its return, may make a great deal of sense to parents. Additional information processing and psychobiologically-based explanations of different trauma-related phenomena (e.g., memory mechanisms, dissociation) may also be presented (see, for example, van der Kolk, 1997; Prasad, 2000).

Developmental explanations relevant to construction of expectations and information processing may also be helpful for parents who worry about the risk to their children's sense of connection and their "shattered assumptions" (Janoff-Bulman, 1992) and confusion about meaning. Adopting a developmental perspective, these explanations underscore the role of the traumatic memory in challenging existing generalized expectations about the safety of the world, the risk to oneself, and the dependability of significant others (Herman, 1997; Pynoos et al., 1996). Some of these explanations are presented more fully in Chapter 5.

The Recovery Environment

The lecture should highlight the significance of the recovery environment and the central impact of parents' functioning on children's postdisaster adaptation. The lecturer can offer important guidelines to parents for active recovery-promoting tasks:

1. Organizing and stabilizing the family life, and providing a sense of continuity, protection, control, optimism, and resiliency. This requires that they monitor their own behavior, take charge of maintaining adequate family functioning, reestablish routines, and be responsive to new needs. This may also involve protecting the child from overexposure to media or other re-traumatizing accounts.

2. Being emotionally available to the child and providing warmth, soothing, and support. This includes the willingness to listen to and acknowledge feelings, clarifying that the child's reactions are expected and normal, encouraging the child's questions and addressing them, providing explanations, and sharing their own concerns in a controlled and manageable way.

3. Providing opportunities for the child to resume a sense of agency, identity, control, and competence through the encouragement of familial, peer, or community social or symbolic activities (e.g., volunteering, showing solidarity and affiliating with others, memorializing), and by acknowledging the strengths and resilience of the child and other family members.

4. Developing sensitive ways of communicating with the child in regard to the emotionally upsetting memories, in order to correct misperceptions and to decrease anxious avoidance. This includes both verbal interactions,

as well as the use of various indirect media such as play, story, and art activity.

5. Attending to signs of distress and symptoms that the child develops in reaction to the traumatic event, and finding ways to offer relief and problem-solve with the child. Problem solving should be based on creatively achieving a balance between acceptance of the child's experienced difficulties and thus the need to make temporary allowances for them on the one hand, and the expectation that the child will return to normal functioning and thus must make some attempt toward gradually resuming coping efforts on the other hand.

Continued Monitoring of the Child's Long-Term Adjustment

The lecture should underscore the need for continued parental monitoring of their children, especially those children considered to be at high risk for developing more persistent disorders. The lecturer should clarify factors associated with a higher risk, especially those related to exposure, intensity of initial reaction to trauma, and individual and familial history and vulnerabilities. Symptoms that require focused assessment and interventions should be defined as those that include elements that do not remit with the passage of time, and which inhibit recovery, such as instances of pervasive, generalized, uncontrollable distress that interferes with rewarding human contact and with necessary functioning, and leads to a negative self-perception. Inasmuch as the term PTSD has gained such popularity in the media, this term should be briefly clarified for parents.

Information Regarding Resources

The lecturer should provide information regarding mental health and other available community resources for future consultation and referral for evaluation and treatment. A handout with the relevant agency names, contact person, address and telephone information and specialization, can be made available at the end of the meeting. Some parents may feel the need at the end of the informative presentation to consult the lecturer individually about their child. Therefore, the crisis team should prearrange the possibility for individual consultation following the assembly with school personnel and school-related mental health professionals.

Integrating Small Groups into the Large-Group Parent Assembly

The suggestions and recommendations made during the large-group assembly cannot always be easily adopted and applied by parents due to their own emotional upset, and the challenge of handling a rather new situation with the child. Some parents need to vent and clarify their feelings and anxieties before they can engage in helping behaviors with their children. The regulation of parental feelings can best be achieved in a small group situation with other parents who share the same, or similar, experiences and difficulties. In our experience, following a crisis, most parents find small discussion groups in a school setting to be an engaging, helpful, and non-stigmatic experience. Therefore, in planning the large-group assembly, the crisis team should allow time for subsequent small-group discussion. This can be achieved by breaking up the group into separate classrooms at the end of the assembly, usually according to the children's grade or class belonging. Alternatively, parents may be divided into smaller groups for a planned activity as part of the large group forum; each small group then reports back to the larger forum as part of the assembly's feedback and closure. At times, at the end of the assembly meeting, parents may be given the option of signing up for small-group meetings to be held on other dates. This is recommended especially when a considerable number of parents appear psychologically distressed, and in need of continuous support due to limited resources, or other high- risk characteristics, such as repeated trauma.

Encouraging Parental Prosocial Involvement

The invitation to parents to become actively involved, by volunteering to help others and perform specific tasks in coordination with the PTA, aims not only to benefit the school but also the parents themselves. Trauma interventionists have widely recognized the beneficial impact of prosocial activity to one's sense of coping and mastery, as well as the sense of solidarity and belongingness to the community. For example, in one parent assembly in a Jerusalem school following a terrorist suicide-bombing that killed the school guard while he was off duty, the parents expressed anxiety about their children's vulnerable security and about the traumatic effect of the symbolic death of the students' protective figure. To feel more involved and gain a sense of more control, the PTA with the support of the families organized various initiatives to provide material, social, and psychological assistance to the late school guard's family. They also raised money to build a playground in the schoolyard to commemorate him and, together with the school, held a moving memorial ceremony when the playground was dedicated.

SMALL-GROUP TRAUMA-RELATED WORK
WITH PARENTS

Small-group work with parents during the first few weeks after a disaster, usually at the recovery phase, may take different forms and attend to different parental needs, depending on the specific event and the characteristics of the parent group. It may place more central emphasis on the parent as an individual, or alternatively, on his or her parenting role. The group format may vary from a single session to a series of meetings.

A small-group intervention may be particularly appropriate for working with linguistically or culturally diverse parents in crisis (Esquivel, 1998). These parents may feel more comfortable in a group setting where they are free to listen and share as much as they want, rather than in an individual session with a mental health professional, which requires more active, continuous conversation and disclosure. When parents do not speak the dominant language it is important to find a group leader, or an assistant to the group leader, who speaks the language of the minority group. Participation in a small group may further help these parents become acquainted with other parents, lessening their sense of isolation due to language or cultural barriers.

The main objective of the small-group meeting or meetings comprises parental empowerment. Various means and techniques may promote this objective. As elaborated below, the intervention usually involves a process of group sharing of experiences and emotions; some focused work on accessing inner resources and solving common problems; and some skills training to help children process their traumatic experience. In order for these objectives to be achieved the group leader(s) must at the outset raise the issue of the safety of the group, and have members agree to respect the confidentiality of the group discussions.

Due to the heightened emotional state of the participants and the crisis-intervention nature of the work it is advisable to have two facilitators lead a group. This format contributes to the sensitivity and effectiveness of the group work and to the psychological well being of the leaders, who can use each other for their own debriefing at the end of the meetings. The leaders may come from any of the helping professions (psychologists, psychiatrists, social workers, counselors, or nurses) but must have training and experience in group work (preferably with parents) and in crisis intervention.

Small-Group Experiential Sharing

Parents may find it beneficial to share with others their personal experience during the traumatic event, and to vent their concerns and worries. The discovery that others are undergoing similar emotional experiences may produce a calming and validating effect. The experiential sharing process may combine educational and psychological elements of debriefing (Dunning, 1990). The educational debriefing model emphasizes sharing of experiences as part of learning about typical and accepted reactions to trauma, whereas the psychological debriefing model underscores ventilation of feelings, experiential reviewing, and emotional sharing. Moreover, the debriefing focuses not only on parents' reactions, but also on children's reactions and on changes in familial relational patterns as a result of the trauma. Parents may feel reassured to hear about similarities and contrasts between their own children's responses and those of other children. Parents may also feel relieved to learn about the widespread frequency of their own postdisaster behavior patterns, such as their need to meticulously monitor their children's whereabouts. The group discussion may also sensitize parents to their more idiosyncratic, unhelpful tendencies such as overprotection, denial, and avoidance. For example, parents may learn that they have talked much less than others to their children about the traumatic experience, and have not been aware of some evolving class occurrences and dynamics.

Nevertheless, caution must be exercised in allowing open sharing of feelings in a group. Without active monitoring by the group leaders, emotional sharing may become an overwhelming experience in a group of highly affected parents. Group leaders must be accepting and empathic to the participants' heightened emotional expressions and must normalize them. However, leaders must also keep the group's emotional atmosphere in check, so as to avoid further demoralization and re-traumatization by group contagion. This is especially pertinent in instances where a sense of helplessness and hopelessness prevails, or when detailed morbid contents of a recounted traumatic incident become too disturbing for group participants. When emotions in the group become too distressing, group leaders should gradually lead the participants to focus more on coping efforts. This shift in focus can be accomplished in a number of ways, such as highlighting the group's role as a helping context for joint problem solving, or leading the group members through a process of self-empowerment through experiential exercises. Creative symbolic activity through artistic expression, writing, or drama therapy may also serve the leaders well in addressing extreme affects (Lahad, 1999).

Joint Problem Solving

Similar concerns shared by a number of parents may lead to a process of group problem solving. In this process, parents who were successful in coping with their own problems, their child's behavioral problem, or family difficulties can "offer their advice" to parents who are still struggling with a similar difficulty. Advice from other parents is frequently more acceptable than advice from experts (Gordon et al, 1999).

When most group members share a mutual concern, they can engage in finding a solution based on their mutual resources as a group. For example, after the death of a student in a suicide bomb explosion on a Jerusalem bus, parents decided to deal with their own, as well as their children's, anxieties about future terrorist threats on public transportation, by organizing a temporary large-scale carpool for driving the children to school and back. In another small group, following a terrorist incident on a downtown Jerusalem street, parents faced a mutual problem: A number of their children had developed avoidance behavior and refused to approach the downtown area. Considering this avoidance to be quite dysfunctional because of the school's downtown location, parents decided on a gradual exposure plan to be carried out together by small groups of parents and their children, exposing them to enjoyable activities in the area (e.g. shopping together, going to the movies or a restaurant).

Parent Empowerment

The salutogenic model that we advocated in Chapter 2 especially suits interventions with caregivers and parents, because it compels them to devote energy toward boosting empowerment and health both within themselves as well as in their children. The group leader may invite participants to share their successful ways of coping with the present disaster, especially how they tap their inner strengths and social resources. Alternatively, parents may be invited to reflect upon a past crisis and how they coped with it. Two major techniques may prove helpful to group leaders in their efforts to empower parents: a coping resources list and guided imagery exercises.

A Coping Resources List

To increase parents' awareness to a wide range of potential personal resources, the leader can present the group with a predesigned list of possible resources and then ask the participants to organize their responses in reference to the list, using guiding questions (see below). This may be implemented in writing or via open interviews with willing participants. The group leader must clarify to the participants that individuals need not use all possible resources on the list, but rather should become cognizant of the ones that they currently use spontaneously, and of those that they may wish to try using in the future.

The list we suggest borrows from the ideas of Lazarus' "multimodal psychotherapy" (1997), and from Lahad and his colleagues (2000), but modifies and expands these further, to suit coping with trauma. Lazarus focused on seven core modalities summed up as the acronym BASIC ID (Behavior, Affect, Sensation, Imagery, Cognition, Interpersonal, and Drugs). It served as the basis of a broad-spectrum, short-term, group crisis intervention following the release of hostages held in 1977 by members of a Muslim sect at three locations in Washington, DC (Sank, 1979).

Along similar lines, Lahad and his colleagues (2000) developed an integrative multimodal coping enhancement program for children in a war zone in Israel organized around BASIC Ph modalities (Beliefs, Affect, Social, Imagination, Cognition, and Physiology). The Israeli Ministry of Education accepted a similar program (Ayalon, 1998) for use in the state educational system. This manualized program was used extensively in schools in northern border communities, exposed to repeated "near miss" missile and terrorist attacks. Both programs have been used in Israel as preparatory guidance programs as well as following large-scale disasters.

Our suggested acronym **BASICS PhD B-ORN** represents the 11 components of our suggested coping resources list, as follows:

Beliefs and values that one experiences as meaningful or as a part of one's identity

Affects that one can experience, express, and modulate (e.g., withholding crying until reaching a safe place)

Sensations that can be augmented or controlled through various sensory inputs (e.g., relaxing by listening to music)

Imagination, altered states of consciousness, creative thinking, and expressiveness (e.g., the ability to meditate, lose oneself in a book, use artistic expression)

Cognitive abilities such as problem-solving skills or original ideas

Social or interpersonal ties, skills, and resources (e.g., having good friends and being able to ask for their help)

Physiology – exercise, sleep, and relaxation

Drive – motivational level, persistence, and determination in pursuing desired goals

Behavior-Organization – the ability to take action and implement changes, or a course of action, upon making a decision

Reflective ability – the ability to think about experiences from different perspectives

Narrative – the ability to integrate experiences into a meaningful coherent story.

In general, parents can be asked to examine their own utilization of each of these resources at two intervals, both during the crisis and afterwards. However, the first eight of these coping resources (BASICS PhD) may be activated very shortly after a traumatic experience, whereas the last three (B-ORN) usually require some time to activate. Therefore, the latter components should be approached more tentatively if implementing a small-group intervention soon after the traumatic experience, and should be presented more as a challenge and an agenda for the future. The group leader can invite participants to reflect on the following (or similar) questions pertaining to the role of these 11 systems in their coping with the traumatic event:

- *The belief system*: Which beliefs, values and convictions helped you cope?
- *The affective system*: Which feelings were aroused, expressed, or modulated? How were they helpful to you?
- *The sensation system*: How did you use your sensory apparatus?

- *The imagination system*: Which means of imaginary distancing, distraction, humor, artistic expression, etc. were helpful to you?
- *The cognitive system*: What kind of information, discussion, self-talk, or problem solving was helpful?
- *The social relatedness system*: Which social skills and who and what in your social environment proved helpful, and how?
- *The physiological system*: Which physical activities were helpful – sports, relaxation, sleep?
- *The drive system*: How did you enlist and sustain your energy and strength?
- *The behavioral-organization and regulatory system*: How did you restructure your life in safer, more meaningful ways?
- *The self-reflective system*: How can you rethink and see a new perspective on the incident, yourself, and others involved? How does that change the meaning of your experience?
- *The narrative system*: How can you integrate the trauma experience into the story of your life, your legacy and identity, your growth? What inspiration or meaning does the story add to your life, to your future goals? What would you want future generations to know about the sources of your agency, strength, vitality, and faith? What contributions do family, culture, community, and history make to these resources?

The discovery of one's resources for successful coping through self-reflection and sharing with the group holds significant potential empowering impact. Listening to other parents' ways of coping may also become a source of modeling and inspiration for adopting additional coping ideas and techniques. Following the discussion of their own resources, parents may be directed to observe their children and use the same conceptualization of resources to identify their child's habitual modes of successful coping.

Other group exercises may include an invitation to imagine the future, or the time when recovery is achieved, and charting in imagination the road to that aspired future time. We have used and further developed in our work with groups following traumatic events one such exercise named "A bridge over troubled water" (Ayalon & Lahad, 2000). The leader invites participants to close their eyes and imagine a bridge between yesterday (the day before the trauma) and tomorrow (the future). Participants are asked to examine such details as the materials composing the bridge, its location and length, the view at each end, how difficulty it is to walk across it. Group members are guided to enrich their imagined journey through additional questions, such as: What is in the bag you are carrying with you? Who is walking with you? Whom do you meet along the way and what do they say to you? Who is waiting for you on the other side?

These questions elicit much symbolic processing as to future potentials and resources that may be helpful in countering feelings of being "stuck," lonely, and insecure. The participants are gently re-oriented at the end of this part of the exercise towards returning from their somewhat dissociated state to the group situation. Paper and crayons are distributed and they are then asked to make a drawing of their bridge. The group members may then be guided towards sharing their bridge story in pairs. Volunteers may be encouraged to share and explore their associations to the fantasy material, with the help of the group leaders in front of the group. Other group members may be encouraged to share with the group their gains from listening to the presenters, but they can also remain silent and experience and process these in a silent, latent fashion.

Parents' Skills Acquisition

Salmon and Bryant (2002) pointed out children's developmental limitations in appraising and coping with their traumatic experience and in initiating discussion about it. They proposed that the significant adults in the child's life, usually the parents, need to support the child in this process. This support requires parents to employ a range of skills like being able to talk about the experience when the child initiates discussion; initiating conversation with the child at appropriate times; correcting misconceptions the child might have; accurately interpreting the child's behavior; and helping the child to label and manage feelings. Joseph (1994) clarified that the support required varies from one child to another. It may include concrete support such as extra time with the parent or an additional night-light, or affective and educational support such as encouragement to express feelings, help in interpreting emotions, and normalization of feelings and reactions.

Although many parents may already possess some or most of the afore-mentioned skills, others may need help in acquiring, strengthening, or practicing their skills in times of stress. Skills training within regular practice of parent counseling, and especially in crisis situations, is often conducted through individual guidance of parents (e.g., Klingman, 1993); however, small groups often provide a more economical setting, especially at times of limited resources such as following a mass disaster. The group format also holds the added benefits of offering opportunities to practice skills while confronting a variety of reactions through role-playing by different group members, and to observe and learn skills from others outside the parental unit.

Group meetings that target various skills should contain both an educational didactic component and a practice component through role-playing. The group leader should encourage sharing and analyzing of both successful experiences, whereby participants applied specific learned skills, and also of unsuccessful experiences, whereby parents encountered difficulties in applying skills or in obtaining cooperative responses from their children. Homework assignments concerning a specific skill may be given to encourage application and refinement of skills, and feedback may be brought back for further group discussion.

We believe no rigid universal skills curriculum can be outlined that would suit the particular needs of a specific small group facing a particular traumatic event. Nevertheless, we next offer some elaboration on several skills that we often find relevant to parents following a traumatic event, including observation and interpretation, communication, and problem solving.

Observational Skills

Often, children communicate their feelings and needs to their parents indirectly, via play and other symbolic activities. Pretending to be a witch or a policeman bringing thieves to prison may reveal anger and guilt feelings. A child may play out fears of destruction and abandonment through aggressive and destructive scenes. Parents who are preoccupied by their own concerns often remain unaware of these communications, which can open a window for parents into the child's inner feelings and thoughts. Teaching parents the skill of becoming participant-observers of such play, especially for younger children, allows the child an opportunity to feel "listened to" and to act out frightening emotions under the soothing and validating influence of the presence of an involved, caring parent. Taking notes on play observations and learning to understand the child's possible messages (whether in the group meetings or in individual guidance sessions) may give parents an opportunity to identify neglected needs and misconceptions of the child, which can then be addressed at appropriate opportunities by the parent.

The widely used filial therapy model (Watts & Broaddus, 2002) not only trains parents in these child observation skills, but also comprises a viable therapeutic intervention for a variety of physical and emotional problems in children. The model promotes positive parent-child interaction and child adjustment and also seems useful for parents of diverse cultural backgrounds (Sweeney & Skurja, 2001). The model encourages parents to conduct regular play sessions with their children, and to employ major techniques used by play therapists. This includes creating special conditions for the sessions, which allow privacy and paying exclusive attention to the child. A "therapeutic" structure is also emphasized, involving a pre-set time, length, and place for the sessions, and the availability of expressive and creative play materials. The training of the parents is conducted, individually or in a group format, through didactic discussions of the principles of sensitive communication with children, as well as through supervision of actual (or videotaped) parent-child play sessions. The parents are trained to follow the child's lead, to be accepting, patient, non-directive, and non-judgmental. The parents learn how to show their interest in the child's actions, feelings, and thoughts through non verbal means (eye contact, physical proximity, facial affect) as well as verbal ones. In particular, they are trained to use "reflection" of the child's communications and to show empathy to the communicated feelings.

The following example demonstrates the benefits of observing and attending to children's messages in play and other symbolic activities, as well as the secondary preventive role of the small-group setting. In a small post-trauma parent group that had received instruction in child observation techniques, one couple brought to the group a description of their kindergarten-age child's activity and play following the traumatic incident that had affected all the residents of their West Bank village in Israel. In that incident, a unit of terrorists had infiltrated the village and entered a number of homes, shooting randomly at residents. The home of the family under discussion was not attacked, but their neighbors suffered grave casualties. In the family at hand, the father had rushed out to join the rescue forces, and the mother locked up the house and hid with her children as they listened to the sounds of gunfire nearby. The parents reported that their son's play at home involved repeated angry fighting and punishing (throwing into jail) of the father play figure. They also reported that in everyday situations, both at home and in kindergarten, the boy would practice climbing up to sit on windowsills and trying to jump out of windows regardless of their dangerous distance from the ground.

In the parent group, exploration of possible meanings for the child's symbolic activities led to the idea that the boy was trying to communicate his anger at his father, for what he had experienced as being abandoned. He was also practicing self-reliant ways of escaping peril. At the same time, he seemed to be calling for his parents to protect him. These tentative understandings helped the parents initiate a new level of communication with the child. The father could empathize with the boy and accept his anger at him, but could then also move ahead to help the child correct his distorted ideas about the father's whereabouts during the incident. Learning that the father was watching and guarding the home from the outside granted the child great relief.

Attentive and systematic observation of older children's behavior may teach parents much about their child's way of coping with a traumatic experience. The group leader can guide parents to look for changes in the child's everyday conduct and to try to comprehend their meaning. For example, close observation of a child's daily activities may uncover a previously unnoticed pattern whereby the child is avoiding reminders of the disaster. Observational monitoring may reveal to the parents the extent to which the child is utilizing inner and outer resources (vis-à-vis the aforementioned list), for example, the child's use of physical outlets such as exercise for the release of tension or the degree to which the child uses peers to gain support, via telephone conversations and social visits. Likewise, parents can attend to the child's use of various means to process the trauma, such as artistic symbolic expressions (e.g., music making, drawing, writing) and informational cognitive pursuits to make sense out of the experience and reduce anxiety, such as "researching" what happened, asking questions, or offering ideas for problem solving through political or security means. The information gleaned from observations may foster parents' efforts to join and communicate with the child through the child's preferred mode of coping, for example by taking interest in the "research."

Communication Skills

Parents often need help in maintaining a communicative stance that shows interest and caring, without becoming intrusive and impatient. The practice of *reflective statements* (e.g., "You look kind of sad") and *"I" messages* (e.g., "I am really willing to listen if you are ready to share") frequently enables parents to accept their child's response or lack of response, and to continue reaching out. The group leader can also clarify that parents who share their own thoughts or feelings with the child without "demanding" an immediate response, or parents who talk to each other about their experience in the passive presence of the child (without overwhelming the child) in fact thereby non-intrusively invite their child to communicate.

Children are often able to communicate more easily when they spend time engaging in an activity with the parent. Shared activities such as gardening, shopping, watching television, cooking, and hiking may not only promote a feeling of return to normalcy but also offer a relaxed atmosphere conducive to spontaneous significant communication. For some youngsters, engaging in a family project such as creating a storybook together (Hanney & Kozlowska, 2002) that contains pictures, newspaper clippings, and written statements may furnish an easier path toward communication than does direct verbal conversation about the traumatic event.

Parents can be helped to develop sensitivity to the child's symbolic and indirect communications expressed through new behaviors. For example, a child may repeatedly call the parents under different pretexts when they are away from home, or may prepare gifts for the parents, time after time, when they go out. Parents who recognize these communications can find a quiet time to initiate a conversation about the child's anxieties about the parents' safety.

Problem-Solving Skills

At times, being supportive and understanding of a child's difficulty does not suffice to help the child overcome that difficulty. School refusal and sleep problems are common examples. Small-group settings offer an opportunity to teach parents how to combine empathic understanding with expectations for coping. Principles of strategic interventions may be helpful in encouraging parents to think creatively about how to deliver this dual message regarding the child's different problems. As an example, in the wake of a traumatic incident, one boy insisted that he could only fall asleep in his parents' bed, and the parents felt that they had to accommodate the child's request. They were also advised, by the group leader, to ask their son to first lie down every night for a few minutes in his own bed, so as not to forget how it felt, in preparation for his return to it. This intervention combined an accommodation to the child's unusual request with symbolic behavior that reflected an expectation for change. Moreover, by introducing an element that created an *ordeal*, this comprised a paradoxical intervention that increased the likelihood of prompt abandonment of the symptom. After all, with time, it may prove more comfortable to remain in one's own bed.

Many parents require assistance in learning strategies for solving problems together with their children, through the clarification of goals and difficulties, and designing a gradual coping plan. Knowledge of cognitive-behavioral techniques (Dattilio & Freeman, 2000; Graham, 1998) may be particularly advantageous in helping children deal with fears through desensitization, and in reinforcing active coping behaviors by systematic attention and recognition of the importance of advancing through small behavioral steps. Thus, to address school refusal, for instance, the parent may construct a gradual plan for returning to school, with the support of the parent's delineated, decreasing timed presence.

After practicing cognitive-behavioral skills in the group, parents can become agents for teaching their children self-monitoring, identification of distorted and unrealistic cognitions, relaxation techniques, thought stopping, and self-instruction and self-reinforcement. A more detailed description of cognitive-behavioral techniques is provided in Chapter 14 on the treatment of PTSD.

Other helpful problem-solving techniques can be drawn from the narrative approach (White & Epston, 1991), which views people as experts on their own lives, and sees problems as separate from people. Techniques such as "externalizing the problem" and looking for "unique outcomes" can enrich parents' repertoire and render them more competent. In working on issues of fears and anxieties, for example, the child may be invited to draw "fear" and give it a name, to think of ways fear affects the child's life, to identify instances when fear takes over, and to recognize ways and circumstances wherein the child can overcome fear's hold.

MULTIPLE FAMILY DISCUSSION GROUPS

We have so far presented models of working with parents that supplement the preventive work carried out, in parallel with their children in school. A more integrative model, which broadens the focus of the intervention to include whole families in a group, may lend itself for use with families following traumatic events. Multiple Family Discussion Groups (MFDG) haves been found effective with various populations such as those with chronic illness, schizophrenia, and learning disabilities (Stern, 2002). Gordon et al. (1999) found that such groups, initiated by an experienced mental health professional in schools and other community settings, offer some unique contributions to empowering children and their families. These groups can offer the children a sense of cohesion through participation with their families in adverse times. Witnessing the children and adults in other families as they express their feelings and disclose family difficulties can help children articulate their own feelings and can contribute to validating and normalizing them.

Gordon et al. (1999) stressed that clinicians working with families in a disaster setting, or following an emergency, need to apply a family crisis model of therapy. This involves structuring at the outset and clarifying the number of sessions and the group's objectives. The objectives should specify the educational and supportive nature of the group and its focus on the crisis and its impact on the children, in the context of the family. The facilitators need to concentrate on identifying and prioritizing the family's problems, identifying its strengths, and mobilizing family members to use them. To maximize the limited contact with the family, the practitioner should provide immediate, clear, and useful advice about the identified distressing problem.

Leading multifamily groups requires the availability of two facilitators, who possess special skills, as they need to engage adults and children at the same time; regulate the pace of the group, and accommodate the focus and the level of discussion and the choice of techniques to fit diverse needs. This format is not recommended for families in which the level of anxiety, confusion or upset displayed by the parents is high. These parents need to regulate themselves before they can constructively communicate with their children. Multifamily groups may be a beneficial format at a later stage of the recovery process, such as around anniversary dates and rituals, offering families an opportunity to gain a perspective on the traumatic event and to further process the event and its implications for their present life and their future as individual families and a community.

Chapter 14

Assessment and Treatment of Trauma-Related Disorders in Children: A Tertiary Prevention Perspective

A s recalled in Chapter 11, the major aims of school-based tertiary pre-vention comprise facilitating the academic and social reintegration into school of children who underwent hospitalization, loss, maladjust-ment, and/or treatment. Yet, systemic efforts at reintegration may at times prove unsuccessful or insufficient for some students who continue, over the long range, to exhibit trauma-related psychological problems, demon-strate a delayed trauma reaction, or show unfavorable developmental changes. This chapter addresses a range of school-based interventions that are both therapeutic, as they are designed to alleviate the distress of stu-dents, but are also designed to play a preventive role in following and counteracting developmental deficits and mental health hazards to high-risk students. The chapter focuses on school-based follow ups, and on school-based group interventions. These can be seen as falling within the continuum between the realms of tertiary prevention and of therapy.

CONCEPTUAL ISSUES IN THE ASSESSMENT OF LONG-TERM EFFECTS OF TRAUMA ON CHILDREN AND IMPLICATIONS FOR INTERVENTION

Most children exposed to traumatic events react with some signs of dis-tress or unusual behavior; yet, by and large, these reactions are transient and wane within a few weeks. Primary and secondary preventive inter-ventions such as those outlined in this book may support this recovery process. Some children's symptoms, however, do not remit and even worsen with the passage of time. These symptoms often fit a clinical diagnosis of PTSD or other trauma-related disorders such as anxiety or depressive disorders. This chapter deals with issues pertaining to the period beyond the first month after the traumatic event, during the recovery stage. We address here the identification and treatment of children who exhibit moderate to severe symptoms of PTSD, anxiety disorder, and depressive disorders, as well as those showing subclinical pictures of PTSD and more general signs of distress and maladaptive functioning (such as somatic complaints, increased aggressiveness, increased dependency, regressive behaviors, decline in school functioning). These children often exhibit a more intense initial reaction to the traumatic event than do their peers, although in some children delayed posttraumatic responses become evident.

Although the literature has focused heavily on the risk for PTSD, we suggest the adoption of a wider developmental psychopathology perspective in assessment and in intervention. This perspective implies the involvement of therapists in addressing obstacles hindering developmental progression and transitions, within an integrative preventive and therapeutic approach. Our emphasis lies on maximizing the therapist's utilization of the resources in the natural systems involved in children's lives: the school system and the family system, as well as additional community systems.

CRITERIA FOR PTSD IN CHILDREN: A CRITICAL EXAMINATION

PTSD refers to the development of a characteristic set of symptoms following exposure to a particularly severe stressor. The relatively recent growing awareness of the relevance of this adult diagnosis for children led in 1994 to some adaptations for children in the *DSM-IV* criteria (American Psychiatric Association, 1994). We described the *DSM-IV* criteria in detail in Chapter 5. The applicability of a PTSD diagnosis for children has attracted much controversy (e.g., Ronen, 2002) between those willing to define certain childhood responses to trauma as a psychiatric disorder and their opponents who view children's responses to trauma as a "normal" reaction to an abnormal situation.

Acknowledgments of the possibility that some children do develop PTSD seem much more prevalent in the recent research literature. However, voices in the literature continue to express definite dissatisfaction and criticisms regarding the diagnostic criteria for childhood PTSD. Most trauma specialists today consider the *DSM-IV* guidelines (American Psychiatric Association, 1994) to be "a work in progress" vis-à-vis children. Yule (2001), for example, described the *DSM-IV* diagnosis as very "adult-o-centric," arguing that some of the *DSM-IV* symptoms (e.g., emotional numbing) are developmentally inappropriate for younger children. He further maintained that lower age correlated with less appropriate *DSM-IV* criteria. Other trauma specialists have voiced similar criticisms regarding the insensitivity of the available criteria to the effects of trauma on young children (AACAP, 1998). Terr (1985) suggested a list of additional PTSD features that she maintained to be different for children in comparison to adults. For example, children do not usually evidence the massive repression or unexpected visual flashbacks that characterize adults, but do demonstrate a dramatic time skew.

Scheeringa and his colleagues (Scheeringa, Zeanah, Drell, and Larrieu, 1995; Scheeringa & Zeanah, 2001) suggested some accommodations and changes in the use of PTSD criteria for children under the age of 6 years, based on their research findings. For example, young children may manifest hyperarousal as somatic complaints and may have difficulty reporting on numbness and avoidance. These researchers recommended adjusting the items in the avoidance/numbing category for children as follows: constriction of play, social withdrawal, restricted range of affect, and loss of acquired developmental skills. Additional criticism has focused on the number of symptoms from each category required to make a PTSD diagnosis in children (AACAP, 1998). Scheeringa and his colleagues suggested that a requirement of only one symptom in the avoidance/numbing category instead of the *DSM-IV*'s 3-symptom requirement (American Psychiatric Association, 1994) would provide a more valid algorithm for identifying PTSD in young children. They further recommended adding a category incorporating young children's most common posttraumatic symptoms, namely: loss of developmental skills, new aggression, new separation anxiety, and new unrelated fears.

It seems that as the professional debate continues about how accurately the *DSM-IV* criteria (American Psychiatric Association, 1994) describe childhood PTSD, these criteria should not become the sole basis for offering therapeutic services to children who do not manage to overcome the effects of the trauma with time.

AN EXPANDED VIEW OF POSTTRAUMATIC ADAPTATION AND PSYCHOPATHOLOGY

In line with our emphasis on prevention, we believe that when dealing with children in the aftermath of traumatic events, focus should lie on ensuring the successful progression of developmental processes. Researchers who work within the attachment theory paradigm (Wright et al., 1997) continually highlight the long-term effects of trauma on children's development. Therefore, the mere use of a classificatory psychopathological approach, which delineates the number and type of symptoms, will not suffice because it disregards the overall quality of the child's adaptation. Child assessment must consider children's progress in the ability to relate to the traumatic event without excessive avoidance and distress, as well as advances in children's resumption of ordinary life and ability to invest in and enjoy routine activities. Patterns that should be considered worrisome include:

- Negative qualitative changes and regressions in the child's relationships with significant others
- A significant deterioration in the child's level of social or academic functioning
- An increase in the level of experienced distress, or a decrease in the level of energy invested in age-related challenges
- The emergence of maladaptive coping patterns, especially of a rigid quality (i.e., avoidance, depression) or of an intense and deregulated nature (angry outbursts, somatic complaints)

This more general emphasis on the developmental implications of traumatic events, rather than on specific symptoms, corresponds with Saltzman, Pynoos, Layne, Steinberg, and Aisenberg (2001) developmental model of childhood traumatic stress. This model underlines not only acute posttraumatic reactions and comorbid reactions including depression, anxiety, and somatic symptoms, but also failure of developmental expectations and guilt, shame, and blame of others. Saltzman and his colleagues particularly emphasize the need to consider the impact of traumatic stress on "proximal development," that is, the level of potential development that can be achieved by a child beyond his or her independent problem-solving activity, by the child's collaboration with others. This includes the achievement of developmental tasks that formulate the ontogenesis of developmental competencies, and the negotiation of developmental transitions. In evaluating risk factors, Saltzman, Pynoos, Layne, Steinberg, and Aisenberg (2002) advocated considering not only aspects of the traumatic experience itself, but also a range of psychological and socio-environmental risk and protective factors related to the pretrauma, peritrauma, and posttrauma ecologies. These entail, for example, the presence of continuous trauma and loss reminders, trauma-related stresses and adversities associated with changes in the child's support system, and the child's history and characteristics. This approach focuses squarely on targeting those factors that cause continuous stress (Layne et al., 2001) and on supporting natural recovery processes rather than merely treating individual symptoms (Shalev, 2002). Farwell and Cole (2001–2002) similarly advocated that assessment and intervention with children exposed to the trauma of war and political violence should therefore incorporate the sociopolitical community as a significant context.

Although some children showing significant symptoms and impairment recover over time without formal intervention, currently no reliable predictors exist to estimate which individual cases will show persistent symptomatology (Cohen et al., 2000). Limited current evidence on PTSD concerning the validity of diagnostic procedures, its natural course, and the effect of specific treatments (Salmon & Bryant, 2002; Ryan & Needham, 2001) indicate a tertiary prevention focus. Indeed, the AACAP (1998) recommended offering treatment to children with symptoms severe enough to impair their functioning in any important domain, whether or not they meet strict PTSD diagnostic criteria according to the *DSM-IV* (American Psychiatric Association, 1994). Similarly, Shalev (2002) suggested that serious disruption in functioning and evidence of factors that inhibit recovery should be used as indications for intervention, rather than observed or reported symptoms. This approach reflects the growing unease in the literature with the risks of a narrow emphasis on the child's PTSD symptoms alone as criteria for intervention.

SCHOOL-BASED ASSESSMENT OF CHILDREN WITH PTSD OR OTHER TRAUMA-RELATED DIFFICULTIES

A preplanned infrastructure should provide continuity of care that supports mechanisms of natural recovery, minimizes stigma, and prevents the possible overburdening of mental health services at times of trauma. This set of care systems for children following disaster includes families, schools (teachers, the school's crisis intervention team), community institutions (collaborating clinical agencies, educational leadership, churches, clubs), peers, neighbors, and more. This infrastructure must aim to identify and treat those children who are most severely affected by the trauma, in the least stigmatizing contexts, and in the most cost-effective manner. School-based interventions are usually least stigmatizing, especially when offered in a group format and when brief in duration. Therefore, our following discussion will focus mainly on these school-integrated identification and treatment approaches. Children and families who find the school setting stigmatizing, however, should be offered other treatment options. We will now outline school-based practices, which are aimed at identifying children who need further therapeutic help to ensure their developmental progress, and to reduce their suffering. We will first examine practices that can be integrated in the ongoing operation of the school and the roles of its various staff members. We will then focus on the more specific practices of psychologists and psychiatrists, who work in collaboration with the school to carry out individual assessments and make recommendations for therapeutic interventions.

IDENTIFYING CHILDREN IN NEED OF THERAPEUTIC INTERVENTION

Following the intense primary preventive interventions of the first few weeks after the trauma, we suggest that schools implement several methods to continue to monitor and strengthen children's adaptation, and to identify those students who require more careful evaluation and focused intensive intervention. To deliver diagnostic and therapeutic services optimally, schools should maintain an ongoing collaborative relationship with a mental health agency, including referral and collaboration procedures. This collaboration can assist the school in planning and implementing a range of prevention, assessment, and treatment methods. As elaborated below, screening methods may encompass periodic group discussions and creative activities; PTSD-related education of school personnel and parents; preparation of a list of at-risk children for follow up; and proactive mass screening.

Periodic Group Discussions and Creative Activities

As a follow-up of the initial primary and secondary preventive interventions around trauma, described in the previous chapters, the school should conduct periodic group discussions and creative activities with children in their classrooms. The most relevant timings of these activities are the one-month, three-month, six-month, and yearly anniversaries of the trauma, and following similar new or related events (another disaster, the capturing or trial of the terrorists, etc.). These times offer an opportunity to explore with children their process of adaptation, explore new perspectives on the trauma, talk about the effect of new trauma reminders, and reflect upon the significance of the anniversary dates, or the new occurrences. This exploration may be conducted via group discussions, or structured expressive art activities. A member of the school's mental health team may moderate these discussions or, alternatively, serve as a support to trained teachers in leading these activities with their students. Observation of the children's reactions, products, and behaviors may provide significant information with regard to children's progress and difficulties in processing the trauma. Additionally, these activities may include an educative component validating the continuing existence of posttraumatic difficulties for some children, and informing children about the availability of helpful interventions. Students may be offered various means of contacting the school's mental health professionals for further help: sending a note, using a "walk-in" hour, calling, etc.

PTSD-Related Education of School Personnel and Parents

Education in regard to PTSD and related long-term reactions following trauma becomes especially useful after the first month following the trauma. It can be achieved through dissemination of written materials to school personnel, an in-service workshop for teachers, and a lecture for interested parents. Parents and teachers who wish to discuss their concerns about a particular child should have easy access to consultation with a mental health professional in the school.

Preparation of a List of At-Risk Children for Follow Up

The school's mental health team, in collaboration with the relevant school personnel, should prepare a list of children whom they consider to be at risk for posttraumatic difficulties. To prepare this list, the team should tap available cumulative information about the child's life history, personality characteristics, and family characteristics, as well as new information on the child's trauma experience, losses, and consequent changes in the child's and family's functioning. In addition, the team should consider the child's initial reactions to the trauma and level of participation in the initial preventive group processing. Informal periodical follow-up of these children through teacher reports, parent reports, classroom observations, and direct interactions with the child may help determine the need for more systematic evaluation.

Proactive-Screening

Mass screening tools can be used for proactive screening of all children in the school system to locate posttraumatic psychopathology and difficulties. Usually, community-based clinical agencies initiate such screenings after augmentation of their services and resources in the months following the trauma in order to deliver both school-based and clinic-based services for affected children and their families. At times, screenings may be conducted as part of a research -based intervention project introduced later (Chemtob, Nakashima & Carlson, 2002). Prior to the screening process, the responsible agency should gain the collaboration of school personnel and parents to reduce the anxiety that screening may provoke in some children and some adults in their natural ecosystems. Indeed, following the September 11 attacks, many parents in the New York City downtown area shared with us their anxiety about PTSD screenings conducted in the school system. Similarly, in the continuously shelled neighborhood of Gilo, in Jerusalem, some children who underwent screening became very defensive about the significance of their reported reactions to a PTSD questionnaire. Special caution must be taken to avoid presenting the results of the screening as a diagnosis, but rather to present them as a first step in a more complex evaluation process involving multiple sources of information (as outlined below in this chapter).

The introduction of proactive mass screening of students in the months or even years after a traumatic event may help school systems that experience burnout in attending to their students' needs. In situations of recurrent traumatic events in Israel during the second Palestinian uprising beginning in September 2000, like repeated shelling episodes in Jerusalem's Gilo neighborhood or frequent terrorist incidents in the West Bank settlements, all systems of care – educational, psychological, and familial – are engaged in managing consecutive crisis interventions. Little energy remains for monitoring the ongoing adjustment of children affected by prior traumas. The recent introduction of trauma treatment projects in Israel and centers, such as the Israel Center for the Treatment of Psychotrauma in Jerusalem, supported by the UJA-Federation of New York (since 2002), seems beneficial in supplementing the regular resources of the overburdened educational and mental health systems. The same argument may apply for systems that, prior to a single traumatic event, were overburdened by the familial and social problems with which their students came to school. Thus, in the aftermath of the WTC tragedy, it is only through the introduction of new resources, and coordinated trauma-focused interventions, via the Children's Mental Health Alliance (see: http//www.cmhalliance.org), that the many mental health needs of children could be addressed in the New York City school system.

PTSD ASSESSMENT TOOLS AND PROCEDURES

Although the school psychologists, or the clinicians of a collaborating agency, are usually responsible for the diagnosis of post- traumatic disorders in children, these professionals' diagnostic work involves inputs from school personnel, and parents. Most trauma specialists recommend a multi-modal and multi-person approach to assessment of PTSD in children (AACAP, 1998; Salmon & Bryant 2002: Yule, 2001). This involves both conducting interviews as well as obtaining standardized assessment data from multiple sources: the child, the parents, and significant others like teachers. A multi-person approach addresses the reliability limitations of single-source data. Parents' reports sometimes minimize children's PTSD symptoms. Teachers and other adults are often unaware of symptoms that manifest themselves only at home, like sleep disturbances. Children's cognitive, self-reflective, and linguistic abilities limit their ability to self-report on symptoms such as avoidance and numbing. Phelps, McCart, and Davies (2002) found that young people exhibited a defensive test-taking approach characterized by denial of stress-related symptoms on self-report measures, particularly when the youth were experiencing affective blunting associated with PTSD. Ronen (2002) advocated careful scrutiny of the child's understanding of the language and the scales when using self-report measures, and supplementing these measures with some observations of nonverbal creative or play activity.

The literature focusing on the clinical assessment of PTSD in children is rather limited. Relatively few validated, published, *DSM-IV*-based (American Psychiatric Association, 1994) measures have been specifically designed to diagnose PTSD in children. New self- and parent-report instruments have been developed in recent years. However, data on their psychometric properties remains limited, and none can yet be considered optimal at this stage (AACAP, 1998; Drake, Bush and van Gorp, 2001). Among the self-report measures considered most promising and most relevant to mass traumatic events and disasters are the following: the *Child's Posttraumatic Stress Reaction Index (CPTS-RI)* developed by Frederick, Pynoos, and Nader (1992); the *Trauma Symptom Checklist for Children (TSCC)* developed by Briere (1996); and the *Child PTSD Symptom Scale (CPSS)* developed by Foa, Johnson, Feeny, and Treadwell (2001). For more information on these inventories and their psychometric properties, as well as others that include self-report and parent-report versions, we refer the reader to the National Center for PTSD website (www.ncptsd.org); Drake et al. (2001); and the AACAP (1998).

PTSD Interviews and Evaluation Considerations

Perrin, Smith, and Yule (2000) maintained that *DSM-IV*-based (American Psychiatric Association, 1994) self-report measures can be used to screen for PTSD, anxiety disorder, and depressive disorder in children over 7 years of age but cannot substitute for a clinical interview. Accurate assessment of PTSD requires a face-to-face semi-structured interview, to be conducted separately with the child and with the parents. For the parent interview, Perrin et al. suggested gathering information beyond the child's symptoms and current functioning, such as information on the child's developmental history and adjustment, family history and problems, and parental reactions to the trauma.

Ronen (2002) advocated that, following the data collection, the clinician's assessment of the need for intervention should involve three elements. First, the clinician should examine the extent to which the child's behavior meets PTSD criteria. Second, the clinician should evaluate the child's behaviors vis-à-vis normal development and typical problems that children exhibit at that age in the child's environment. Third, the clinician should focus on the developmental tasks and skills relevant to the child's stage of development, which are most likely to be affected by the trauma. These comprehensive considerations can reveal not only the appropriateness of a PTSD diagnosis, but also, more importantly, whether the child is suffering and needs help in overcoming his or her distress.

Many clinicians use semi-structured interviews designed to assess PTSD in children and adolescents. None of the available semi-structured interviews has been extensively evaluated psychometrically with regard to a clinical PTSD diagnosis based on the *DSM-IV* (American Psychiatric Association, 1994). These interviews are time consuming and require much clinical skill. Some interview schedules, which seem promising in terms of accumulating psychometric data, and which are administered both to the child and to the parents, include: the *Clinician-Administered PTSD Scale*

for Children and Adolescents for DSM-IV (CAPS-CA) developed by the
National Center for PTSD and researchers from the University of California at Los Angeles (UCLA) (Nader et al., 1996) and the *Children's PTSD
Inventory (CPTSDI)* developed by Saigh et al. (2000). Detailed descriptions
of these interviews and their psychometric properties data can be found
in Drake et al. (2001) and the AACAP (1998).

While these interview schedules attempt to elicit direct information in
relation to post- traumatic symptoms, some other child interview
procedures have been developed to access unconscious materials, through
means that encourage projection. These means include projective tests,
projective interviews, and play assessments.

The Use of Projective Tests, Activities, and Interviews

Trauma specialists (e.g., Drake et al., 2001; Zeidner, Klingman, & Itskovitz,
1993) have highlighted the advantage of projective techniques in evaluating children for PTSD because such techniques allow access to both conscious and unconscious aspects of the child's functioning. These specialists
advocated the use of well-known and child-friendly projective tests, like
the Children's Apperception Test, the Thematic Apperception Test, and
the Rorschach.

Inasmuch as many children exhibit difficulties in responding to direct
questioning, either because of their age or because of emotional inhibitions
in talking about the traumatic experience, Nader and Pynoos (1991) advocated the use of a draw-a-picture and tell-a-story exercise, in either an
individual, or a classroom group setting, in the aftermath of a traumatic
event. This procedure can serve both as a psychological first-aid intervention as well as a screening for posttraumatic stress and other symptomatic reactions. Assessment of the data elicited by this exercise focuses on
the embedded perceptual aspects of the trauma and on the central action
and intervention fantasies that may indicate blaming, self-blame, and guilt.
This provides an assessment of the child's current level of stress and may
assist in monitoring progress in therapy, but does not provide in itself a
diagnosis of PTSD.

The Use of Play for Assessment

Nader and Pynoos (1991) suggested actively encouraging the child to
engage in play. The therapist's active interventions and the availability of
toys that can represent aspects of the traumatic event will facilitate the
play. The active interventions should be designed to expand children's
exploration of their subjective experience and to restore ego functioning,
thus serving both an evaluative and therapeutic function.

Terr (1983, 1990) has conducted extensive ongoing observations of the
play of a group of traumatized children, whom she followed for several

years after they had been kidnapped. She described a number of characteristics of posttraumatic play that distinguish it from ordinary play. Posttraumatic play entails many compulsive repetitions with the same
outcomes and also fails to relieve the child's anxiety. Such play is literal,
with no elaborations, and uses simple defenses like identification with the
aggressor, displacement, undoing, transforming passive into active, and
denial in latency. Neither "corrective reworking" nor "working- through"
appear. Play is ritualistic, constricted, joyless, and even morbid. It lacks
the spontaneity and animation characterizing the play of non-traumat-
ized children.

SCHOOL-BASED THERAPEUTIC INTERVENTIONS FOR CHILDREN WITH PTSD OR OTHER TRAUMA-RELATED DIFFICULTIES

School-based therapies for children boast a range of configurations and
theoretical approaches, as well as several essential components.

Structural Aspects of Intervention

Despite the growing number of controlled treatment outcome studies for
PTSD in children, existing data from such studies remains insufficient and
does not establish the clear advantage of one treatment over another
(Pfefferbaum, 1997; Ryan & Needham, 2001; Shepperd, 2000). This state-
of-the-art substantiates the need for the comprehensive, multimodal, and
multidimensional treatment of children suffering from PTSD and other
trauma-related disorders (AACAP, 1998; Woodcock, 2000). Comprehensive treatment addresses various symptoms and difficulties and relates to
various adversities (such as trauma, losses, and bereavement). The therapeutic work is multidimensional as it draws from various theoretical
approaches and involves many modalities. Different structural modalities
for intervention may include components of individual, group, and family
therapy either simultaneously or at different stages of the intervention.
Research evidence supports the benefits of establishing school-based programs for the treatment of children suffering from PTSD (Chemtob, Nakashima & Carlson, 2002). Whereas most trauma specialists have highlighted
the major contribution of including one or more parent-directed components in the child's treatment plan (AACAP, 1998), in effect, many intervention projects neglect parental involvement, instead focusing on direct
work with the children (March et al., 1998; Chemtob, Nakashima & Carlson, 2002).

Reported interventions vary in client selection criteria. Most include
children and adolescents who report postdisaster symptoms (Chemtob,

Nakashima & Hamada, 2002; Goenjian et al., 1997; Saltzman et al., 2001) rather than full-blown PTSD (Chemtob, Nakashima & Carlson, 2002; March et al., 1998). The duration of the interventions and frequency of sessions also vary greatly, from three weekly sessions (e.g., Chemtob, Nakashima & Carlson, 2002) to monthly sessions throughout a full academic year (e.g., Galante & Foa, 1986). Duration and frequency depend on the needs of the affected children, the requirements of a particular treatment protocol, and the accessibility of financial resources and professional availability. In our opinion, a pulsed (intermittent) schedule for interventions provides the optimal structure, especially when resources are limited. The introduction of periodic interventions at strategic points is conducive to readjustments that anticipate and address the course of recovery, with a focus on more specifically identified needs and intractable problems at different times (Chemtob, Nakashima & Hamada, 2002; Pfefferbaum, 1997).

Theoretical Basis for Interventions

Several therapeutic approaches may serve as the basis for school-based interventions targeting children with PTSD: cognitive-behavioral therapies, eye movement and desensitization reprocessing, psychodynamic psychotherapies, narrative and constructivist therapies, family therapy, and integrative approaches. We will first consider the major theoretical tenets of two of these approaches, which are most relevant to school-based group interventions, yet differ markedly in their orientations.

Trauma-Focused Cognitive-Behavioral Therapies (CBT)

Despite the limited literature on controlled treatments, growing evidence from outcome studies for childhood PTSD supports the effectiveness of CBT in individual, parent, or group formats (AACAP, 1998; Perrin et al., 2000). CBT derives from cognitive theories, such as Foa, Steketee, and Rothbaum's (1989) proposed information processing theory of PTSD (see Chapter 5). It is assumed that circuits of "fear networks"" must be activated in a prolonged manner to permit habituation of anxiety and to weaken associations with threat. The formation of adaptive schemata depends on corrective information that is incompatible with the previous harm-related schema. Thus, CBT focuses on a process of prolonged exposure, habituation of anxiety, and correction of distorted information

Perrin et al. (2000) described a basic model of CBT for children with PTSD. Following assessment and the establishment of a therapeutic alliance with the child and the parents, treatment addresses four major components:

1. Education and preparation: focusing on the normalization of the

child's reactions and on providing a rationale for treatment, including mutual specific goal setting.

2. Coping skills development: including the teaching of relaxation, positive self-talk, thought stopping, and problem solving techniques.

3. Exposure: including "imaginal" exposure, which involves encouraging the child to recall the event in detail, and to reexperience all relevant thoughts and emotions. The therapist questions the child about the most difficult aspects of the traumatic experience. Monitoring the child's level of distress during this process, and using relaxation techniques when distress increases, ensures that the disturbing emotions can be mastered rather than magnified. With young children, drawings are often added to the verbal account. To gradually reduce avoidance behavior, the therapist assigns homework that encourages "in vivo" exposure to avoided trauma-related reminders and activities.

4. Termination and relapse prevention: including summarizing what has been learned and the gains made. Additionally, the therapist asks the child to identify potentially stressful future situations and to remember appropriate coping techniques.

Criticisms of the cognitive behavioral approach with children have focused mainly on the risks elicited by the exposure component. Clearly, exposure sessions may be counter productive by including excessive gruesome details, by being too short to process the strong evoked emotions, and by leaving children in a heightened state of arousal thus sensitizing them rather than helping to habituate anxiety. Some of the limitations of CBT relate more to age and coping style. Young children may be incapable of abstract discussions of emotions and thought processes. They may be unable to imagine traumatic material, follow relaxation procedures, or tolerate exposure (Saigh, Yule & Inamdar, 1996). Avoidant children may resist cooperation with instructions to confront the avoided thoughts and images (Phillips, 2000). Furthermore, persistent talking about traumatic events to children who are very embarrassed or highly resistant may in fact worsen symptoms (AACAP, 1998). Addressing traumatic issues indirectly through the use of art (e.g., drama, drawings, play) may be helpful in such cases.

In our experience in situations of ongoing and repeated traumatic incidents, exposure techniques must be used in a carefully monitored way, as the traumatic event cannot be processed as a past danger. Although the facts of the event and its emotional impact must be acknowledged, more symbolic and indirect means of processing of thoughts and emotions (drawing, writing, rituals) are often more useful. Furthermore, in-vivo exposure is often perceived by therapists and clients as realistically potentially dangerous. Narrative techniques, which emphasize the meaning of survival and suffering, may be more helpful in these situations.

Narrative and Constructivist Therapies for Traumatized Children

Narrative therapy derives from the post-modern premise that people organize their experience through the stories they tell themselves, which then shape their perceptions, feelings, and behaviors. People come to therapy with problem-saturated stories influenced by culture. The narrative approach views people as experts on their own lives and views problems as if they were a separate entity (not inherent in the person) that oppresses the client and the client's family (Nichols & Schwartz, 1998). It assumes that people have many abilities, competencies, values, and commitments that will assist them to reduce the influence of problems on their lives. Narrative therapy involves examining people's problem-saturated life stories, deconstructing them, and then introducing collaborative ways of re-authoring these stories. White (2002) maintained that rather than viewing the pain and symptoms resulting from trauma as psychopathological reactions, they may be viewed as testimony to the cherished purposes for people's lives, their prized values and beliefs, and hopes and moral visions about how things might be in the world.

Given the central role allocated to imaginal exposure in overcoming posttraumatic symptoms in cognitive-behavioral interventions, it is important to note that proponents of the narrative approach take a different position in regard to this practice. Narrative therapists are careful to avoid interventions that might invite the child to reexperience the trauma and its related feelings of powerlessness and helplessness. Although narrative therapists provide ample opportunities for children to express and validate their experiences via the expressive arts, emphasis lies on helping children separate from the problem stories and access more preferred stories (Adams-Westcott & Dobbins, 1997). Thus, initial contact with the children should focus not on the traumatic events, but rather on what the children value in life and on aspects of their lives that are not dominated by the effects of the traumatic events. Experiences in therapy that externalize the problem and its effects will facilitate the process of separating the child from the trauma-dominated story. *Externalizing conversations* employ language or activities to locate the problem outside the person (White & Epston, 1991). With young children, the problem is given a name and is represented in a drawing or some other nonverbal medium, to enable children to demonstrate the effects of past trauma on their lives today. To encourage children to see that these influences do not necessarily have to continue into the future, the therapist should challenge the children to locate experiences that contradict the assumed inevitable power or impact of the trauma, and to acknowledge their own qualities that can support these achievements in overcoming the hold of the trauma. The therapist supports this process of internalizing positive qualities by inviting, either in imagination or in reality, the presence of supportive significant adults who can nurture the children, empower their positive self-references, and celebrate their achievements.

The narrative approach focuses on the ability to explore different possible meanings of the traumatic events, and on adopting those that are most validating and empowering to the survivor. This "re-authoring" approach further focuses on the contribution of the validation of these meanings through the support of significant others and wider communities. Shalif and Leibler (2002) demonstrated how attention to language and the power of ideology, religion, and community support could play a central role in deconstructing the negative meaning of "trauma," in countering the experience of psychopathology, and in supporting the potential for growth.

Ronen (1996, 2002) applied a similar but much more structured *constructivist* approach to traumatized children. The *cognitive-constructivist* approach emphasizes the child's developmentally-linked abilities for personal monitoring, meaning-making, and awareness of the processes involved and their functions. Ronen recommended that children should be helped to understand and accept traumatic events as part of life, and to give these events new meaning, which can generate better coping and potential growth and maturation. She further advocated challenging and empowering children to open themselves up to the world and to new experiences.

Some possible implications of the narrative therapy approach for mental health professionals in the school system involve a de-emphasis on the utilization of diagnostic evaluations and structured interventions. Narrative therapy may be useful for systems with a limited motivation or objections for using exposure-based interventions (such as CBT), or those exposed to ongoing repeated traumatic events.

An Integrative View

We believe that therapeutic intervention should not be grounded in only one theoretical approach. Consensus holds that a more optimal approach will integrate elements from cognitive-behavioral, psychodynamic, narrative, and family therapies (March et al., 1998). These elements may either be blended or selected to suit children's age, symptoms, and coping style as well as contextual and cultural factors (Shepperd, 2000; Woodcock, 2000). Likewise, although CBT is considered safe and effective in treating PTSD symptoms in general, its effectiveness depends on the child's cognitive abstract and reflective abilities, motivation, and level of arousal and avoidance. Therefore, the introduction of psychodynamic play and other symbolic modalities may better suit the needs of some children rather than do direct discussions of traumatic material (Phillips, 2000; Ryan & Needham, 2001). Likewise, it is advisable to take an integrative stance in relation to school and clinic-based interventions. For example, school-based interventions may comprise the ideal setting for correcting misperceptions and for encouraging normalization and recovery, but may not suit the discussion of revenge fantasies. In addition, school-based interventions may not suffice for some children, who will require more individualized and intensive clinical work to tackle specific disturbing thoughts and images (March et al., 1998; Pfefferbaum, 1997).

Despite the many differences in theoretical explanations for PTSD and the diversity of intervention techniques, strong consensus seems to exist in the field as to the essential components of treatment for children with PTSD (AACAP, 1998). These components include, first, the reduction of anxiety and anxiety-related symptoms. This component usually involves teaching children specific *stress management* techniques. The therapist often couples stress management with a direct exploration of the trauma experience, although for some children this seems to arouse too much anxiety, and some approaches (e.g., the narrative approach) de-emphasize this component.

Second, in the main, therapists recognize the importance of adopting a wider perspective on the traumatic events' pervasive effects on how victims view themselves and the world. This issue requires therapeutic exploration, challenging, and correction of inaccurate attributions regarding the trauma. Additionally, treatment must attempt to transform children's self-concept from victim to survivor, replacing the experience of helplessness with an acknowledgement of their own agency and resources in coping with the trauma. Third, these goals can only be achieved in a setting that provides a safe context for sharing painful and overwhelming experiences, as well as intense feelings like rage, revenge, and guilt (Pfefferbaum, 1997).

School-Based Group Interventions for PTSD

Therapeutic group work can provide an effective treatment option for children and adolescents with, or with a predisposition toward PTSD. Researchers described group work as more economical yet at least equally effective in comparison to individual treatment, in at least two thirds of the cases (Glass & Thompson, 2000). Thus, group counseling can also serve as a screening intervention to identify high-risk children who should be referred for additional individual diagnosis and therapy (Cohen et al., 2000).

For latency age children, the small peer group comprises a natural, familiar setting. Group therapy in a school setting may be optimal for schoolchildren who have experienced a common trauma (Cohen et al., 2000). The natural school setting, familiar peer group format, and shared experiences prevent most traumatized children from feeling singled out or stigmatized. The group setting may help avoidant children feel less pressured to speak yet more involved in the latent processing of their traumatic experiences, in comparison to an individual setting. Most children in a group eventually find the appropriate words to express what has happened to them. The group setting creates opportunities for the use of various experiential and creative modes of processing traumatic memories and feelings, through such activities as games, drama, brainstorming, art projects, and writing. These activities often become much richer and emotionally powerful in a group context. Furthermore, sharing feelings with peers who have undergone the same experience seems to allow children to open up and not only to receive genuine support and empathy, but also to give it to others. This may strengthen their sense of efficacy.

Glass and Thompson (2000) offered an overview of the issues that should be covered in groups of children and adolescents who suffer from PTSD symptoms. These include:

1. Emotional expression: Allowing an opportunity for expressing emotions, such as anger, grief, anxiety, guilt, numbness, relief, and so on, and an opportunity for these emotions to be validated and accepted.
2. Narrative recounting: Describing and reconstructing the traumatic experience, verifying facts, and acknowledging and understanding its personal significance.
3. Constructive exploration: Exploring past losses and traumatic events, and their possible connection to the present experience.
4. Specific symptoms: Employing cognitive behavioral techniques such as relaxation to cope with symptoms related to anxiety.
5. Problem solving: Discovering ways to deal with everyday difficulties by using brainstorming in the group, using one's past experiences, and finding out about possible sources of support.
6. Addressing future plans: Encouraging setting goals and making realistic plans at a time when the sense of future is obscured by the traumatic event.

Group leaders must keep in mind the risk of re-traumatizing some participants by overexposing them to the trauma accounts of their peers. The leaders must therefore balance exposure experiences with relaxation techniques and empowerment exercises, and monitor the emotional responses of all group members while a single participant is actively processing his or her trauma experience. It is possible to integrate individual and family interventions in order to channel the processing of individual traumatic memories in a more intimate and individualized manner, through such activities as continuous diary writing or sharing with one of the therapists individually. Mannarino, Cohen, and Stubenbort (2002) recommended that the child should share the trauma narrative with the parents in a joint session following adequate preparation in separate meetings.

A number of school-based group programs for the treatment of adolescents exposed to trauma and traumatic loss have been established and evaluated in recent years. These interventions usually targeted postdisaster trauma-related symptoms rather than PTSD (Chemtob, Nakashima & Hamada, 2002; Goenjian et al., 1997; Saltzman et al., 2002). March and his colleagues (1998) targeted schoolchildren who evidenced a primary, full PTSD diagnosis and who had each individually suffered a single traumatic incident. Their intervention consisted of a school-based, group-administered, 18-week cognitive-behavioral psychotherapy protocol for children 10 to 15 years old. This protocol was designed on the basis of a theoretical model integrating the social and biological bases of PTSD with social-learning theory, conditioning theory, and cognitive information processing. Anxiety management training in the program attempted to promote children's habituation to conditioned anxiety using relaxation training. Further elements of training aimed to develop children's skills for coping with disturbing affects and physiological sensations, and included anger control and positive self-talk. Narrative exposure, through each child's sharing of his or her trauma story with the group, allowed opportunities for training in undesirable response prevention, for normalizing responses, and for introducing necessary revisions of trauma-induced distortions and misattributions. The group facilitators assigned in vivo exposure as homework, to gradually overcome avoidant everyday behavior, with the aide of the acquired anxiety management skills.

The program emerged as safe, effective, and durable in alleviating PTSD symptoms, as well as symptoms of depression and anxiety. March and his colleagues (1998) claimed that their program's main gains occurred through children's enhanced sense of predictability and controllability, which may have resulted from both the cognitive training and the exposure components. However, their program did not take advantage of its school-based setting by including parents or teachers.

The UCLA Trauma Psychiatry Program also developed a school-based manualized trauma- and grief-focused group psychotherapy intervention for symptomatic adolescents following a disaster or loss (Saltzman et al., 2001). The UCLA program was implemented with some modifications in Armenia after an earthquake (Goenjian et al., 1997), in post-war Bosnia (Layne et al., 2001), and in a high-crime area of Southern California (Saltzman, Pynoos, et al., 2001), demonstrating much promise according to effectiveness evaluations. The program was designed as a 16- to 20-week intervention, preceded by thorough screening of each participant's symptomatology and by matching of participants to groups according to the type (trauma or loss experience) and severity of exposure. The program entailed a combination of group psychotherapy, adjunctive individual and family therapy, and assessment of improvement. In Armenia, the intervention was shortened to 6 weeks, combining group and individual sessions (Goenjian et al., 1997). The main foci of the program are:

1. *The traumatic experience.* These group interventions, like similar ones presented above, aim to increase tolerance and improve regulation

of trauma-related material utilizing psychoeducation and normalization of posttraumatic reactions, narrative construction including
exploration of the worst traumatic moments, cognitive restructuring
of the experience, and so on.

2. *Trauma and loss reminders.* This involves efforts to promote effective
   coping with distressing reminders, and using reminders to explore
   the personal meaning of the traumatic event.

3. *Secondary adversities.* This focus addresses the life changes and current
   difficulties that are related to the trauma and loss, and the development of coping and problem-solving strategies to contend with them.

4. *Grief.* This unique focus attempts to deal with the complexity of traumatic bereavement by reducing the traumatic avoidance to free up
   psychological resources for the grieving process. Interventions
   include psychoedcation and construction of a non-traumatic mental
   image of the deceased, and dealing with loss-related emotions such
   as shame and guilt. Parents are invited to a group meeting to participate in sharing loss-related feelings and memories of the deceased.

5. *Developmental impact.* This focus, also rather unique to this program,
   attempts to identify the adolescents' missed developmental opportunities and their current difficulties in functioning, and to initiate
   more desirable developmental progression and prosocial adjustment.

Whereas the UCLA program seems most suitable for the treatment of
adolescents, Chemtob, Nakashima, and Hamada (2002) developed and
evaluated an integrative psychosocial intervention for postdisaster trauma
symptoms in elementary school children. The intervention followed a
manualized protocol and consisted of four sessions, either individual or
group. Resembling the aforementioned protocols to a large extent, these
sessions focused on safety and helplessness, loss, mobilizing competence,
issues of anger, and ending and going forward. However, unlike the other
interventions, Chemtob et al.'s treatment included a standard box of play
and art materials and incorporated experiential activities designed to elicit
reflections relevant to each session. Despite its brevity, the intervention
was reported to be effective in reducing disaster-related symptoms in children 2 years after a hurricane disaster. Interestingly, although the group
and individual treatments did not differ in efficacy, fewer children
dropped out of the group treatment. This finding strengthens our conten-
tion about the possible relative advantages of group school-based interventions for posttraumatic problems.

School-Based Group Programs for the Treatment of Depression and Anxiety Disorders

A number of field-tested comprehensive interventions exist for children
and youth exhibiting depression. Although these programs have not been

developed in the context of dealing with the aftermath of traumatic events, their structure and techniques lend themselves readily to such use. Merrell (2001) described four such programs deriving from a cognitive-behavioral approach. One program, the adolescent coping with depression course (CWD-A) seems most relevant to our focus on school interventions. This highly structured psychoeducational program for the treatment of adolescent depression included 16 small-group 2-hour sessions and additional sessions for parents. The program incorporated explanations, modeling and practice, and individual assignments regarding the application of new skills. These skills encompassed self-observation, positive thinking, disputing irrational thinking, relaxation, communication, and problem solving.

Merrell (2001) also described five programs for the treatment of anxiety. The 18-session "Coping Cat" program, for example, for groups of schoolchildren aged 9 and up, entailed two phases. In the first phase, group facilitators taught children to identify the somatic, cognitive, and behavioral components of anxiety. The second phase involved application of new skills for overcoming anxiety, including self-monitoring, identification of distorted and unrealistic cognitions, relaxation, and self-instruction and self-reinforcement.

These programs targeting depression or anxiety possess a much narrower focus in comparison to the previously described interventions targeting posttraumatic symptoms. Such school-based programs, tailored to the specific dynamics and symptoms of children previously diagnosed as suffering from either depression or anxiety disorder, can be implemented, as an adjunct to the programs for children suffering from PTSD.

SCHOOL-BASED INDIVIDUAL INTERVENTIONS

Community mental health agencies usually offer individual and family interventions for children who continue to suffer from posttraumatic difficulties beyond the typical recovery period. However, schools sometimes possess the capacity to offer such services, especially if they are short-term or intermittent and if the school can access the necessary resources in terms of trained clinicians, mental health personnel hours, and appropriate physical space. For many children and families, the school location feels more comfortable and less stigmatic than a mental health clinic.

School-Based Eye Movement and Desensitization Reprocessing (EMDR)

This client-paced exposure treatment that incorporates elements from cognitive-behavioral treatments was developed by Shapiro (1995) and adapted for use with children by Greenwald (2001). Shapiro assumed that through the procedure of inducing sets of eye movements while the client is concentrating on memory-related images, thoughts, and sensations, and concomitantly tracking the back-and-forth hand movements of the therapist, accelerated information processing of dysfunctionally stored traumatic material occurred. Critics of the procedure have called into question the relative contribution of the eye movement procedure to the cognitive interventions that aim to process traumatic memories, suggesting that EMDR constitutes a comprehensive integrative trauma intervention, even without the eye movement procedure. Chemtob, Nakashima, and Carlson (2002) introduced an EMDR intervention through the elementary school system, consisting of 3 sessions of treatment with children who continued to evidence PTSD 3 years after a hurricane disaster. They demonstrated both its short-term and long-term effectiveness in dramatically reducing PTSD symptoms and in more modestly reducing symptoms of depression and anxiety. Although more controlled research is needed to validate its effectiveness and to compare it with that of other intervention programs, the brevity of EMDR intervention and its potential effectiveness may suggest the feasibility of training school-associated therapists in its usage.

School-Based Play Therapy for Traumatized Children

Play therapy has been widely acknowledged as an extremely powerful modality for treating children's problems (Chazan, 2002; Drewes, 2001). For children who suffer the pain of trauma, play offers a chance to use their imagination, creativity, and problem-solving abilities to modify past experiences and to use new coping strategies.

Most reports of play therapy with traumatized children targeted child abuse and neglect (Gil, 1994), but some applications have targeted other traumatic situations such as accidents, disasters, violence, and terrorism (Webb, 1991, 2002b; Ryan & Needham, 2001). Play therapy is traditionally carried out in clinical settings. Recent developments, however, have increased the feasibility and even advantageousness of conducting play therapy in school settings (Drewes, Carey & Schaefer, 2001). The new development of short-term play therapy models makes this option especially viable (Kaduson & Schaefer, 2000). Nader (2002), for example, suggested the integration of directive play therapy in treating children after incidents of violence in schools. She maintained that a single session, or several sessions when needed, may facilitate the abreactive processing of the traumatic impressions and emotions. The introduction of toy replicas representing aspects of the event, and the therapist's active though sensitive encouragement of the child to process a set of memories and emotions, can expedite the child's resolution of difficult aspects of the traumatic experience.

Short-term Gestalt play therapy comprises another form of directive play therapy that involves creativity and sensitivity on the part of the therapist in order to strengthen the child's sense of self, as a prelude to expressing emotions. Oaklander (2000) demonstrated this approach in her work with grieving children, addressing feelings of confusion, abandonment, guilt, betrayal, shame, responsibility for parents, etc. The therapeutic meetings are intermittent, and parents are invited to participate in at least one meeting.

In contrast to these directive play therapy models, some therapists (e.g., Ryan & Needham, 2001) support a non-directive approach to play therapy with traumatized children. They argue that non-directive models avoid direct confrontation with the trauma itself and thus minimize the risks of strong negative emotional reactions in children with PTSD. Non-directive play therapists respect the child's pace and need for current defenses and uphold a strong belief in children's ability to work optimally on their own issues given favorable conditions. These therapists value symbolic play interventions rather than purely verbal approaches. The model is innovative in its short-term 8-session structure (despite its non-directive nature) and its incorporation of parents.

FAMILY AND PARENT THERAPY

In line with our arguments in previous chapters (Chapters 7 and 13), most trauma specialists espouse the idea that interventions with traumatized children must include their families (AACAP, 1998; Berliner, 1997; Cohen et al., 2000). Most of the reported family therapy work around posttraumatic reactions in children focuses on child abuse, with only rather limited literature describing and evaluating family-based interventions around disasters (Dreman & Cohen, 1982, 1990; Figley, 1998; Klingman, 1992; Reilly, 2002; Terr, 1989). This paucity of models for postdisaster parent counseling and family therapy is surprising given the wider recognition these models have received in different theoretical orientations addressing therapy of childhood disorders. Even within traditional therapeutic approaches (e.g., psychoanalytic), recognition is growing for the benefits of parent therapy as an alternative to direct child treatment (Jacobs & Wachs, 2002). Parent therapy involves therapeutic work with the parents alone, directed at ameliorating the child's problems through changes induced in the parent-child relationships, as a result of changes in the way the parents perceive, experience, and understand the child. CBT applications have also indicated that parental inclusion in interventions might result in better therapy outcomes (Barrett, Dadds & Rapee, 1996; Mash & Barkley, 1998). Family-centered approaches generally seem two-pronged, focusing on the parenting role and on systemic functioning.

Focus on Parenting Roles

The parenting role focus enlists parents as adjunct change agents to support the child's struggle with posttraumatic problems. This focus is appropriate when the family system remains relatively stable in the aftermath of the trauma and when the parents are coping relatively well emotionally. Parenting role interventions teach parents principles derived from trauma-focused interventions (such as those described earlier in this chapter), including principles of facilitating trauma and grief processing, and problem solving. Such interventions may come in lieu of direct interventions with the child or as an adjunct to individual or group interventions with the child. Additionally, in vivo interventions are carried out in family sessions to facilitate communication between the child and the parents regarding the traumatic experience, and related feelings and cognitions. Gil (1994) introduced play and other expressive techniques into family therapy to improve difficult communication, claiming the particular merits of *family play therapy* for families who treat their children like little adults. This parental supportive focus may be addressed in school-based programs as part of a comprehensive intervention plan for affected children. From our experience, especially in cases of family bereavement, interventions benefit from separate child and parent settings initially, to deal with different issues burdening them and to perform preparatory work for meeting together as a family.

Focus on Family System Functioning

The second family focus, on systemic functioning, is usually addressed in a clinical setting outside the school, but a school mental health professional should maintain contact with the family therapist, to help in collaborative efforts designed to assist the child. This more traditional focus of family therapy involves a more comprehensive intervention within the family system to reduce trauma-induced disruptions in its functioning. Therapeutic work targets systemic postdisaster changes that have affected communication, closeness, flexibility, and problem solving in the different family subsystems (Olson, 1997), as well as role allocation and intergenerational boundaries (Faust, 2001). The introduction of narrative and constructivist elements may empower the family system and help them make sense out of what happened (Figley 1988). Reflection and narrative construction are often enhanced by such activities as creating a family storybook or picture books, especially in families with young children, as detailed by Hanney and Kozlowska (2002).

As mentioned above, when a family participates in a clinic-based intervention and gives its consent, the school should encourage a collaborative relationship with the family therapist, to enhance significant school personnel's tolerance, understanding, and support of the child. This collaboration appears most crucial in special cases of traumatic parental death. For example, family systems may need particular support from schools when issues of loss and foster-parenting are involved. When children lose both parents, the foster-families face complex challenges in integrating the children into their new families, and the school can provide assistance by monitoring and supporting the children's social and academic integration (Dreman & Cohen, 1982). Family therapy can also address step-parent issues that emerge even years after the traumatic loss, when a parent remarries and issues of children's loyalties to the memory of the deceased parent take the form of behavior problems. The school's awareness of these occurrences and collaborative efforts may help ease these crises for children.

Endnote

Throughout this book, we have emphasized a number of messages, some of which may initially appear contradictory, but we hope they gradually became reconciled and integrated for the reader. One such message, supported by our review of the literature, asserts that mass traumatic events challenge the coping systems of those affected and represent a serious mental health risk to children and the adults around them. A related, seemingly contradictory message, based on our professional experiences and some of the reviewed literature, contends that individuals possess impressive abilities for creatively utilizing inner and outer resources to deal with crises, to regain mastery over adverse events, and to even grow psychologically as a result of successful coping with traumatic experiences. We attempted to integrate these two messages by illuminating the essential components of prevention and intervention that aim to concurrently reduce the aforementioned risk while also increasing the likelihood of positive coping, recovery, resilience, and psychological wellness by capitalizing on the strengths of both individuals and their natural support systems. We have advocated a major shift, from a purely medical-clinical model that focuses on individual treatments of those children identified as suffering from a disorder as an outcome of disaster, to multiple emphases on the recovery environment of all the involved children, on preventive efforts within children's natural environments, and on the use of generic principles in handling disasters. These emphases include special attention to the early identification and continuous follow up of high-risk individuals and sub-groups, and to the tailoring of appropriate non-stigmatic interventions for them. It is within this perspective that we have placed the school system as a preferred organizational, social, and professional center for prevention, intervention, and follow up efforts concerning youngsters' coping with traumatic events.

Investors in school preparedness may meet with various difficulties. Thus, we have stressed in this book the benefits that a school system may reap through in-house preparedness and resilience building for meeting everyday crises and challenges, which often lead to a more cohesive and nurturing community.

We have also demonstrated the important central role of the school mental health professionals in this work. Their role, especially that of school psychologists, has undergone significant changes in many systems over the last decade, as schools have begun to increasingly depend on professionals within the school system instead of community mental health professionals for psychological care of children affected by crises (Allen et al., 2002). The growing inclusion of crisis intervention in university curriculum and training, and the continued broadening of the school psychologist's and the school counselor's role definition to include preventive school-wide initiatives for enhancing schools' safety and effectiveness, will hopefully provide further impetus for these professionals' growing involvement and leadership in the area of trauma prevention and crisis intervention.

This change needs to be supported by a policy decision by the professional leadership of the school mental health services and the top educational administration officials. This decision should call for an intensive in-service crisis management training workshop for all psychologists as well as follow up training and supervision. We suggest that such training focus on three major areas:

1. The acquisition of knowledge (theory, research, conceptualizations) about the characteristics of crisis and emergency situations, as well as the distinctive qualities of crisis interventions and the generic principles underlying them.
2. Clarification of personal feelings and attitudes about intervention in crisis situations, internalization of the benefits of prevention and early intervention, and personal empowerment.
3. Experiential development of skills relevant to interventions prior to, during, and in the aftermath of a disaster or crisis. These skills should relate to interventions at the organizational level, the group level, and the individual level.

Although this book does not directly elaborate on training, it offers much of the material needed for such training. In addition to the theoretical and empirical background on disasters, stress responses, and positive responding, we have spelled out the conceptual basis underlying preventative intervention. We have included detailed accounts and examples of the activities carried out by the mental health staff in the roles of educators, consultants, team members, and short term therapists, which illustrate the skills that need to be developed in training. Nevertheless, by advocating training of school mental health professionals for prevention, crisis intervention, and trauma work, we do not imply that they become the "specialists" who directly carry out the necessary interventions. Rather, mental health personnel should disseminate their knowledge with relevant adaptations to teachers, school administration, support staff, parents, and community leaders. Dissemination of knowledge and responsibility is important to create a unifying approach and a "common language," and in order to initiate and develop multisystemic collaborative work. Our detailed model of group work conducted with parents in the aftermath of trauma (see Chapter 13) may serve as a training model that can be adapted for the training of teachers, or of support staff. Such adaptations may require certain modifications that take into account participants' different role demands, existing talents, and expertise. The many examples provided in the book on the rich variety of activities undertaken by teachers (see Chapter 12) can further clarify the specific skills available to teachers, which can be enlisted and used in their newly assumed roles in crisis situations.

In outlining the benefits of a multisystemic approach to trauma, we emphasized its greater psychological impact, professional richness, and cost effectiveness. This approach necessitates clarification, preplanning, and coordination for establishing partnerships and multisystemic collaboration between the different groups constituting the school and its community: teaching staff, school support staff, school administration, school mental health staff, students and parents, regional administration, community mental health agencies, and other community agencies and institutions. Such partnerships allow each group to act as helpers and to be helped when needed. We have demonstrated this chain of helping by describing school-based interventions with parents, aimed at empowering parents to help the students, as well as enlisting parents' resources to help the functioning of the school, in the aftermath of a disaster. Likewise, we have stressed the benefits of the collaboration between community mental health agencies, the school mental health professionals, and teaching staff, especially during the post-recovery period. These benefits allow for comprehensive follow ups, identification of children suffering from posttraumatic reactions, and the delivery of tertiary preventive diagnostic and therapeutic interventions in a non-stigmatic format and setting. The added impetus of the peer group and of families to the process of recovery of those more severely affected by the trauma is also underscored in our presented models of group work in the school setting and coordinated work with school-linked treatments provided elsewhere.

The model we have presented in this book places the teacher in a number of significant roles in times of crises, beyond his or her traditional role as an expert in instruction. Namely, the teacher may become an "educator" (modeling, inspiring, and facilitating positive coping), a significant attachment figure, and a "clinical mediator." Although teachers may initially be reluctant to assume these roles, our repeated experiences attest that with proper training, supervision, and empowerment, teachers may experience much personal and professional growth in taking on these roles. They may learn, together with other school personnel, that helping children under duress often requires no more than small acts of sensitivity, warmth, encouragement, and simple advice shared by the children among themselves or through the adults who care for them. The principles guiding the multisystemic joint work can all be translated into various educational activities in the classroom, whether related to organizing information, introducing daily structure and safety, allowing for expression and processing of inner reactions, or fostering the regulation of behavior through active coping and problem solving. Thus, we approach the school setting as a sort of therapeutic milieu, where the cooperative efforts of schools, families, and community agencies erect a "protective shield" for children against the risks of trauma.

We hope that our accentuation of empowerment, resiliency, strengths, growth, and a positive outlook in coping with adverse events instigates our readers to engage in creatively "translating" the knowledge base and experiences presented in the book into their own disaster preparation efforts and into trauma-focused interventions when adverse events thwart the "basic assumptions" and mental health of the children under their care.

References

Adams-Westcott, J. A. & Dobbins, C. (1997). Listening with your "heart ears" and other ways young people can escape the effects of sexual abuse. In C. Smith & D. Nyland (Eds.), *Narrative therapies with children and adolescents* (pp. 195–220). New York: Guilford Press.

Aguilera, D. C. & Messic, J. M. (1978). *Crisis intervention: Theory and methodology.* St. Louis: Mosby.

Al-Krenawi, A. & Graham, J. R. (2000). Culturally sensitive social work practice with Arab clients in mental health settings. *Health and Social Work, 25,* 9–22.

Al-Krenawi, A., Graham, J. R. & Sehwail, M. A. (2002). Bereavement responses among Palestinian widows, daughters and sons following the Hebron massacre. *Omega: Journal of Death and Dying, 44,* 241–255.

Allen, M., Jerome, A., White, A., Marston, S., Lamb, S., Pope, D., et al. (2002). The preparation of school psychologists for crisis intervention. *Psychology in the Schools, 39,* 427–439.

Almqvist, K. & Brandell-Forsberg, M. (1995). Iranian refugee children in Sweden. *American Journal of Orthopsychiatry, 65,* 225–237.

Alon, N. & Levine Bar-Yoseph, T. (1994). An approach to the treatment of post-traumatic stress disorder (PTSD). In P. Clarkson & M. Pokorny (Eds.), *The handbook of psychotherapy* (pp. 451–469). New York: Routledge.

American Academy of Child and Adolescent Psychiatry. (1998). Practice parameters for the assessment and the treatment of children and adolescents with posttraumatic stress disorder. *Journal of the American Academy of Child and Adolescent Psychiatry, 37*(suppl.10S), 4S-26S.

American Academy of Pediatrics, Work Group on Disasters. (1995). *Psychological issues for children and families in disasters: A guide for the primary care physician.* Retrieved March 7, 2001, from http://www.mentalhealth.org/ publications/allpubs/SMA 95–3022/default.asp.

American Psychiatric Association. (1980). *Diagnostic and statistical manual of mental disorders* (3rd ed.). Washington, DC: Author.

American Psychiatric Association. (1994). *Diagnostic and statistical manual of mental disorders* (4th ed.). Washington, DC: Author.

American Psychiatric Association. (2000). *Diagnostic and statistical manual of mental disorders* (4th ed., text rev.). Washington, DC: Author.

American Red Cross. (2001). *Facing fear: Helping young people deal with terrorism and tragic events.* Falls Church, VA: Author.

Amirkhan, J. H. & Greaves, H. (2003). Sense of coherence and stress: The mechanics of healthy disposition. *Psychology and Health, 18,* 31–62.

Antonovsky, A. (1987). *Unraveling the mystery of health: How people manage stress and stay well.* San Francisco: Jossey-Bass.

203

Antonovsky, A. (1990). Pathways leading to successful coping and health. In M. Rosenbaum (Ed.), *Learned resourcefulness* (pp. 31–52). New York: Springer.

Aptekar, L. & Stoecklin, D. (1997). Children in particularly difficult circumstances. In J. W. Berry, P. R. Dasen & T. S. Saraswathi (Eds.), *Handbook of cross-cultural psychology* (2nd ed., vol. 2, pp. 377–412). Boston: Allyn and Bacon.

Artiss, K. L. (1963). Human behavior under stress: From combat to social psychiatry. *Military Medicine, 128,* 1011–1019.

Arzi, N. B., Solomon, Z. & Dekel, R. (2000). Secondary traumatization among wives of PTSD and post-concussion casualties: Distress, caregiver burden and psychological separation. *Brain-Injury, 14,* 725–736.

Asarnow, J., Glynn, S., Pynoos, R. S., Nahum, J., Guthrie, D., Cantwell, D. P., et al. (1999). When the earth stops shaking: Earthquake sequelae among children diagnosed for pre-earthquake psychopathology. *Journal of the American Academy of Child and Adolescent Psychiatry, 38,* 1016–1023.

Aspinwall, L. G. & Taylor, S. E. (1997). A stitch in time: Self regulation and proactive coping. *Psychological Bulletin, 121,* 417–436.

Ayalon, O. (1998). Community healing for children traumatized by war. *International Review of Psychiatry, 10,* 224–233.

Ayalon, O. & Lahad, M. (2000). *Hayim al hagvul* [Life on the edge]. Kiryat -Tivon, Israel: Nord.

Bandura, A. (1982). Self-efficacy mechanism in human agency. *American Psychologist, 49,* 389–404.

Barnes, M. F. (1998). Understanding the secondary traumatic stress of parents. In C. R. Figley (Ed.), *Burnout in families: The systemic costs of caring* (pp. 75–89). Boca Raton, FL: CRC Press.

Barrett, P. M., Dadds, M. R. & Rapee, M. R. (1996). Family treatment of childhood anxiety: A controlled trial. *Journal of Consulting and Clinical Psychology, 64,* 333–342.

Bartholomew, R. E. & Wessely, S. (2002). Protean nature of mass sociogenic illness: From possessed nuns to chemical and biological terrorism fears. *British Journal of Psychiatry, 180,* 300–306.

Bateson, G. (1972). *Steps to an ecology of mind: Collected essays in anthropology, psychiatry, evolution, and epistemology.* San Francisco: Chandler.

Bat-Zion, N. & Levy-Shiff, R. (1993). Children in war: Stress and coping reactions under the threat of Scud missile attacks and the effect of proximity. In L. A. Leavitt & N. A. Fox (Eds.), *The psychological effects of war and violence on children* (pp. 143–161). Hillsdale, NJ: Lawrence Erlbaum.

Beck, A. & Katcher, A. (1983). *Between pets and people.* New York: Putnum.

Belter, R. W., & Shannon, M. P. (1993). Impact of natural disasters on children and families. In C. F. Saylor, *Children and disasters* (pp. 85–103). New York: Plenum.

Benedek, E. (1979). The child's rights in times of disaster. *Psychiatric Annals, 9,* 58–61.

Benedek, E. P. (1985). Children and disaster: Emerging issues. *Psychiatric Annals, 15,* 168–172.

Bennett, M. J. (2001). *The empathic healer: An endangered species?* New York: Academic Press.

Berk, J. H. (1998). Trauma and resilience during war: A look at the children and humanitarian aid workers of Bosnia. *Psychoanalytic Review, 85,* 639–658.

Berliner, L. (1997). Interventions with children who experienced trauma. In D. Cicchetti & S. L. Toth (Eds.), *Rochester Symposium on Developmental Psychopathology: Vol 8. Developmental perspectives on trauma: Theory, research, and intervention* (pp. 491–514). Rochester, NY: University of Rochester Press.

Berman, S. L., Kurtines, W. M., Silverman, W. K. & Serafini, L. T. (1996). The impact of exposure to crime and violence on urban youth. *American Journal of Orthopsychiatry, 66,* 329–336.

Bevin, T. (1991). Multiple traumas of refugees: Near drowning and witnessing of maternal rape: Case of Sergio, age 9. In N. B. Webb (Ed.), *Play therapy with children in crisis: A casebook for practitioners* (pp. 92–110). New York: Guilford Press.

Bisson, J. I., McFarlane, A. C. & Rose, S. (2000). Psychological debriefing. In E. B. Foa, T. M. Keane & M. J. Friedman (Eds.), *Effective treatments for PTSD* (pp. 39–60). New York: Guilford Press.

Blackwelder, N. L. (1995). Critical incident stress debriefing for school employees. *Dissertation Abstract International,* 56(4), 1192A.

Bleich, A., Dycian, A., Koslowsky, M., Solomon, Z. & Wiener, M. (1992). Psychiatric implications of missile attacks on a civilian population: Israeli lessons from the Persian Gulf War. *Journal of the American Medical Association,* 268, 613–615.

Bolton, D., O' Ryan, D., Udwin, O., Boyle, S. & Yule, W. (2000). The long-term psychological effects of a disaster experienced in adolescence: II. General psychology. *Journal of Child Psychology and Psychiatry and Allied Disciplines,* 41, 513–523.

Bowlby, J. (1961). Processes of mourning. *International Journal of Psycho-Analysis,* 42, 317–340.

Bowlby, J. (1969). *Attachment and Loss:* Vol. 1. Attachment. London: Hogarth Press and the Institute of Psycho-Analysis.

Bowlby, J. (1988). *A Secure Base: Clinical Applications of Attachment Theory.* London: Routledge.

Breslau, N. (1998). Epidemiology of trauma and posttraumatic stress disorder. In R. Yehuda (Ed.), *Psychological trauma* (pp. 1–29). Washington, DC: American Psychiatric Press.

Breton, J. J., Valla, J. P. & Lambert, J. (1993). Industrial disaster and mental health of children and their parents. *Journal of the American Academy of Child and Adolescent Psychiatry,* 32, 438–445.

Breznitz, S. (Ed.). (1983). *The denial of stress.* New York: International Universities Press.

Briere, J. (1996) *Trauma Symptom Checklist for Children.* (TSCC). Odessa, FL: Psychological Assessment Resources.

Brock, S. E. (2002a). Group crisis intervention. In S. E. Brock, P. J. Lazarus & S. R. Jimerson (Eds.), *Best practices in school crisis prevention and intervention* (pp. 385–404). Bethesda, MD: National Association of School Psychologists.

Brock, S. E. (2002b). Identifying individuals at risk for psychological trauma. In S. E. Brock, P. J. Lazarus & S. R. Jimerson (Eds.), *Best practices in school crisis prevention and intervention* (pp. 367–384). Bethesda, MD: National Association of School Psychologists.

Brock, S. E., Lazarus, P. J. & Jimerson, S. R. (Eds.). (2002). *Best practices in school crisis prevention and intervention.* Bethesda, MD: National Association of School Psychologists Publication.

Brock, S. E. & Poland, S. (2002). School crisis preparedness. In S. E. Brock, P. J. Lazarus & S. R. Jimerson (Eds.), *Best practices in school crisis prevention and intervention* (pp. 273–288). Bethesda, MD: National Association of School Psychologists.

Brock, S. E., Sandoval, J. & Lewis, S. (2001). *Preparing for crisis in the schools: A manual for building school crisis response team* (2nd. ed.). New York: Wiley.

Brom, D. & Kleber, R. (1989). Prevention of post-traumatic stress disorder. *Journal of Traumatic Stress,* 2, 335–351.

Brom, D. & Kleber, R. (2000). On coping with trauma and coping with grief: Similarities and differences. In R. Malkinson, S. S. Rubin & E. Witztum (Eds.), *Traumatic and nontraumatic loss and bereavement: Clinical theory and practice* (pp. 41–66). Madison, CT: Psychological Press.

Bronfenbrenner, U. (1979). Contexts of child rearing: Problems and prospects. *American Psychologist,* 34, 844–850.

Brooks, R. B. (2002). Creating nurturing classroom environments: Fostering hope and resiliency as an antidote to violence. In S. E. Brock, P. J. Lazarus & S. R. Jimerson (Eds.), *Best practices in school crisis prevention and intervention* (pp. 61–91). Bethesda, MD: National Association of School Psychologists.

Burnett, J. J. (1998). A strategic approach to managing crisis. *Public Relations Review,* 24, 475–488.

Calhoun, L. G. & Tedeschi, R. G. (1999). *Facilitating posttraumatic growth.* Mahwah, NJ: Lawrence Erlbaum Associates.

Caplan, G. (1964). *Principles of preventive psychiatry.* New York: Basic Books.

Carlier, I. (2000). Critical incident stress debriefing. In A. Y. Shalev, R. Yehuda & A. C. McFarlane (Eds.), *International handbook of human response to trauma* (pp. 379–387). Dordrecht, Netherlands: Kluwer Academic Publishers.

Caspi, A., Bolger, N. & Eckenrode, J. (1987). Linking person and context in the daily stress process. *Journal of Personality and Social Psychology,* 52, 184–195.

Casswell, G. (1997). Learning from the aftermath: The response of mental health workers to a school bus crash. *Clinical Child Psychology and Psychiatry,* 2, 517–523.

Chazan, S. E. (2002). *Profiles of play*. London: Jessica Kingsley.

Chemtob, C. M., Nakashima, J. P. & Carlson, J. G. (2002). Brief treatment for elementary school children with disaster-related posttraumatic stress disorder: A field study. *Journal of Clinical Psychology, 58,* 99–112.

Chemtob, C. M., NaKashima, J. P. & Hamada, R. S. (2002). Psychosocial intervention for postdisaster trauma symptoms in elementary school children: A controlled community field study. *Archives of Pediatrics and Adolescent Medicine, 156,* 211–216.

Cohen, D. (Ed.). (1987). *The power of psychology*. New York: Croom Helm.

Cohen, E. (2000). Shinuim hitnahagutiyim vedarhay hitmodedut shel bnei noar leahar pgiaa bivney shihvatam-Divuah horim [Behavioral changes and coping of adolescents following the loss of class mates- Parental reports]. In A. Klingman, A. Raviv & B. Stein (Eds.), Yeladim bemazavei herum velahatz (pp. 532–540). Jerusalem, Israel: The Psychological and Counseling Service, Ministry of Education.

Cohen, J. A., Berliner, L. & March, J. (2000). Treatment of children and adolescents. In E. B. Foa, T. M. Keane & M. J. Friedman (Eds.), *Effective treatments for PTSD* (pp. 106–138). New York: Guilford Press.

Compas, B. E. & Epping, J. E. (1993). Stress and coping in children and families: Implications for children coping with disaster. In C. F. Saylor (Ed.), *Children and disaster* (pp. 11–28). New York: Plenum Press.

Dattilio, F. M. & Freeman, A. (Eds.). (2000). *Cognitive-behavioral strategies in crisis intervention*. New York: Guilford Press

Davidson, W. B. & Cotter, P. R. (1986). The relationship between sense of communality and subjective well-being: A first look. *Journal of Community Psychology, 19,* 246–253.

DeBellis, M. D. (1997). Posttraumatic stress disorder and acute stress disorder. In R. T. Ammerman & M. Hersen (Eds.), *Handbook of prevention and treatment with children and adolescents: Interventions in the world context* (pp. 455–494). New York: Wiley.

Desivilya, H. S., Gal, R. & Ayalon, O. (1996a). Extent of victimization, traumatic stress symptoms, and adjustment of terrorist assault survivors: A long-term follow-up. *Journal of Traumatic Stress, 9,* 881–889.

Desivilya, H. S., Gal, R. & Ayalon, O. (1996b). Long-term effects of trauma in adolescence: Comparison between survivors of a terrorist attack and control counterparts. *Anxiety, Stress, and Coping, 9,* 135–150.

Dohrty, G. W. (1999). Cross-cultural counseling in disaster [Electronic version]. *The Australian Journal of Disaster and Trauma Studies, 2,* NP.

Drake, E. B., Bush, S. F. & van Gorp, W. G. (2001). Evaluation and assessment of PTSD in children and adolescents. In S. Eth (Ed.), *PTSD in children and adolescents* (pp. 1–30). Washington, DC: American Psychiatric Association.

Dreman, S. & Cohen, E. (1982). Children of victims of terrorist activities: A family approach to dealing with tragedy. *American Journal of Family Therapy, 10,* 39–47.

Dreman, S. & Cohen, E. (1990). Children of victims of terrorism revisited: Integrating individual and family treatment approaches. *American Journal of Orthopsychiatry, 60,* 204–209.

Drewes, A. A. (2001). Developmental considerations in play and play therapy with traumatized children. In A. A. Drewes, L. J. Carey & C. E. Schaefer (Eds.), *School- based play therapy* (pp. 297–314). New York: Wiley.

Drewes, A. A., Carey L. J. & Schaefer C. E. (Eds.). (2001). *School- based play therapy*. New York: Wiley.

Dunning, C. (1990). Mental health seqealae in disaster workers: Prevention and intervention. *International Journal of Mental Health, 19,* 91–103.

Dwairy, M. A. (1998). *Cross-cultural counseling: The Arab-Palestinian case*. New York: Haworth Press.

Dyregrov, A. (1996). Children's participation in rituals. *Bereavement Care, 15,* 2–5.

Egeland, B., Carlson, E. & Sroufe, A. (1993). Resilience as process. *Development and Psychopathology, 5,* 517–528.

Esquivel, G. B. (1998). Group interventions with culturally and linguistically diverse students. In

K. C. Stoiber & T. R. Kratochwill (Eds.), *Handbook of group intervention for children and families* (pp. 252–267). Boston: Allyn & Bacon.

Eth, S. (Ed.). (2001). *PTSD in children and adolescents*. Washington, DC: American Psychiatric Association.

Everly, G. S. (2000a). Pastoral crisis intervention: Toward a definition. *International Journal of Emergency Mental Health, 2*, 69–71.

Everly, G. S. (2000b). The role of pastoral crisis intervention in disasters, terrorism, violence, and other community crisis. *International Journal of Mental Health, 2*, 139–142.

Everly, G. S. & Mitchell, J. T. (1999). *Critical Incident Stress Management (CISM): A new era and standard of care in crisis intervention*. Ellicott City, MD: Chevron.

Everly, G. S. & Mitchell, J. T (2000). The debriefing "controversy" and crisis intervention: A review of lexical and substantive issues. *International Journal of Emergency Mental health, 2*, 211–225.

Eyre, A. (1999). In remembrance: Post-disaster rituals and symbols. *Australian Journal of Emergency Management, 14*, 22–29.

Farwell, N. & Cole, J. B. (2001–2002). Community as a context of healing. *International Journal of Mental Health, 30*, 19–41.

Faust, J. (2001). Post traumatic stress disorder in children and adolescents: Conceptualization and treatment. In H. Orvaschel, J. Faust & M. Hersen (Eds.), *Handbook of conceptualization and treatment of child psychopathology* (pp. 239–265). Amsterdam: Pergamon.

Figley, C. (1988). A five-phase treatment of post-traumatic stress disorder in families. *Journal of Traumatic Stress, 1*, 127–139.

Figley, C. R. (1993). War-related stress and family-centered intervention: American children and the Gulf war. In L. A. Leavitt & N. A. Fox (Eds.), *The psychological effects of war and violence on children* (pp. 339–356). Hillsdale, NJ: Lawrence Erlbaum Associates.

Figley, C. R. (Ed.). (1998). *Burnout in families: The systemic costs of caring*. Boca Raton, FL: CRC Press.

Fleming, S. & Balmer, L. (1996). Bereavement in adolescence. In C. A. Corr & D. E. Balk (Eds.), *Handbook of adolescent death and bereavement* (pp. 139–154). New York: Springer.

Flynn, B. W. (1996, April). *Psychological aspects of terrorism*. Paper presented at the First Harvard Symposium on the Medical Consequences of Terrorism, Boston, MA.

Foa, E. B., Johnson, K. M., Feeny, N. C., Treadwell, K. R. H. (2001). The child PTSD Symptom Scale: A preliminary examination of its psychometric properties. *Journal of community Psychology, 30*, 376–384.

Foa, E. B. & Meadows, E. A. (1997). Psychosocial treatments for posttraumatic stress disorder: A critical review. *Annual Review of Psychology, 48*, 449–480.

Foa, E. B., Steketee, G. & Rothbaum, B. O. (1989). Behavioral/cognitive conceptualization of post traumatic stress disorder. *Behavior Therapy, 20*, 155–176.

Folkman, S. & Lazarus, R. S. (1985). If it changes it must be a process: Study of emotion and coping during three stages of a college examination. *Journal of Personality and Social Psychology, 48*, 150–170.

Fothergill, A., Maestas, E. & Darlington, J. D. (1999). Race, ethnicity and disasters in the US: A review of the literature. *Disaster, 23*, 156–173.

Frederick, C., Pynoos, R. S. & Nader, K. O. (1992). Childhood PTSD Reaction Index (CPTS-RI). Unpublished Manuscript. UCLA.

Freud, A. & Burlingham, D. (1943). *War and Children*. New York: International University Press.

Galante, R. & Foa, D. (1986) An epidemiological study of psychic trauma and treatment effectiveness for children after a natural disaster. *Journal of the American Academy of Child Psychiatry, 25*, 357–363.

Galea, S., Ahern, J., Resnick, H., Kilparick, D., Bucuvalas, M., Gold, J., et al. (2002). Psychological sequelae of the September 11 terrorist attacks in New York City. *The New England Journal of Medicine, 346*, 982–987.

Garbarino, J. (1992) Developmental consequences of living in dangerous and unstable environments: The situation of refugee children. In M. McCallin (Ed.), *The psychological well-being of refugee children: Research, practice and policy issues* (pp. 1–23). Geneva: International Catholic Child Bureau.

Garbarino, J. (1995). Growing up in a socially toxic environment: Life for children and families in the 1990s. In G. B. Melton (Ed.), *The individual, the family, and social good: Personal fulfillment in times of change* (pp. 1–20). Lincoln, NE: University of Nebraska Press.

Gidron, Y. (2002). Posttraumatic stress disorder after terrorist attacks: A review. *Journal of Nervous and Mental Disease, 190,* 118–121.

Gil, E. (1994). *Play in family therapy.* New York: Brunner/ Mazel.

Gillham, J. E., Reivich, K. J. & Shatte, A. J. (2001). Building optimism and preventing depressive symptoms in children. In E. C. Change (Ed.), *Optimism and pessimism: Implication for therapy, research, and practices* (pp. 301–320). Wasington, DC: American Psychological Association.

Ginzburg, K., Solomon, Z. & Bleich, A. (2002). Repressive coping style, acute disorder, and post-traumatic stress disorder after myocardial infarction. *Psychosomatic Medicine, 64,* 748–757.

Gist, R. & Lubin, B. (1999). *Response to disaster: Psychological, community, and ecological approaches.* Philadelphia: Brunner/Mazel.

Glass, D. & Thompson, S. (2000). Therapeutic group work. In K. N. Dwivedi (Ed.), *Post-traumatic stress disorder in children and adolescents* (pp. 163–183). London: Whurr.

Glass, T. A. & Schoch-Spana, M. (2002). Bioterrorism and the people: How to vaccinate a city against panic. *Clinical Infectious Diseases, 34,* 217–223.

Goenjian, A. K., Karayan, I., Pynoos, R. S., Minassian, D., Najarian, L. M., Steinberg, A. M., et al. (1997). Outcome of psychotherapy among early adolescents after trauma. *American Journal of Psychiatry, 154,* 536–542.

Gordon, N. S., Farberow, N. L. & Maida, C. A. (1999). *Children and disasters.* Philadelphia, PA: Brunner/ Mazel.

Graham, P. H. (Ed.). (1998). *Cognitive-behavior therapy for children and families.* New York: Cambridge University Press.

Greenberg, B. S. (1993). Summary and commentary. In B. S. Greenberg & W. Gantz (Eds.), *Desert Storm in the mass media* (pp. 397–436). Chesskill, NJ: Hampton Press.

Greenwald, R. (2000). The trauma orientation and child therapy. In K. N. Dwivedi (Ed.), *Post-traumatic stress disorder in children and adolescents* (pp. 7–24). London: Whurr.

Greenwald, R. (2001). *Eye movement desensitization and reprocessing (EMDR) in child and adolescent psychotherapy.* Northvale, NJ: Jason Aronson.

Gudas, L. J. (1993). Concepts of death and loss in childhood and adolescence: A developmental perspective. In C. F. Saylor (Ed.), *Children and disasters* (pp. 67–84). New York: Plenum Press.

Gurwitch, R. H. & Messenbaugh, A. (2001). *Healing after trauma skills: A manual for professionals, teachers, and families working with children after disaster.* Oklahoma City, OK: Children's Medical Research Foundation.

Gurwitch, R. H., Sitterle, K. A., Young, B. H. & Pfefferbaum, B. (2002). The aftermath of terrorism. In A. M. La Greca, W. K. Silverman, E. Vernberg & M. C. Roberts (Eds.), *Helping children cope with disasters and terrorism* (pp. 327–357). Washington, DC: American Psychological Association.

Gutkin, T. B. (1999). Collaborative versus directive/prescriptive/expert school-based consultation: Reviewing and resolving a false dichotomy. *Journal of School Psychology, 37,* 161–190.

Gutkin, T. B. & Curtis, M. J. (1999). School-based consultation theory and practice: The art and science at indirect service delivery. In C. R. Reynolds & T. B. Gutkin (Eds.), *The handbook of school psychology* (3rd ed., pp. 598–637). New York: Wiley.

Hanney, L. & Kozlowska, K. (2002). Healing traumatized children: Creating illustrated storybooks in family therapy. *Family Process, 41,* 37–65.

Harkness, L. (1993). Transgenerational transmission of war-related trauma. In J. P. Wilson & B. Raphael (Eds.) *International handbook of traumatic stress syndromes* (pp. 635–643). New York: Plenum Press.

Hartman, C. R. & Burgess, A. W. (1993). Information processing of trauma. *Child Abuse and Neglect, 17,* 47–58.

Helping children and adolescents cope with violence and disasters. (n.d). Retrieved September 21, 2003 from http://www.nih.gov/publicat/violence.cfm

Henggeler, S. W., Schenwald, S. K., Bordin, C., Rowland, M. D. & Cunningham, P. B. (1998).

Multisystemic treatment of anti-social behavior in children and adolescents. New York: Guilford Press.

Herman, J. (1997) *Trauma and recovery.* New York: Basic Books.

Hobfoll, S. E. (2001). The influence of cultural, community, and the nested-self in the stress process: Advancing conservation of resources theory. *Applied Psychology: An International Review, 50,* 337–370.

Hobfoll, S. E., Spielberger, C. D., Breznitz, S., Figley, C., Folkman, S., Leppen-Green, B., et al. (1991). War related stress: Addressing the stress of war and other traumatic events. *American Psychologist, 46,* 848–855.

Hodgkinson, P. (2000). Post-traumatic stress disorder. In C. Feltham & I. Horton (Eds.), *Handbook of counselling and psychotherapy* (pp. 502–509). London, UK: Sage.

Holloway, H. C., Norwood, A. E., Fullerton, C. S., Engel, C. C. & Ursano, R. J. (1997). The threat of biological weapons: Prophylaxis and mitigation of psychological and social consequences. *Journal of the American Medical Association, 278,* 425–427.

Horowitz, D. & Lissak, M. (1989). *Trouble in utopia: The overburdened policy of Israel.* New York: State University of New York Press.

Horowitz, M. J. (1976). *Stress response syndromes.* Oxford, UK: Jason Aronson.

Hoven, C. W., Duarte, C. S., Lucas, C. P., Mandell, D. J., Cohen, M., Rosen, C., et al. (2002). *Effects of the World Trade Center attack on NYC public school student: Initial report to the New York City Board of Education.* Columbia University Mailman School of Public Health — New York State Psychiatric Institute and Applied Research and Counseling, LLC, New York City.

Howe, M. L. (1997). Children's memory for traumatic experiences. *Learning and Individual Differences, 9,* 153–174.

Hsu, C . C., Chong, M. Y., Yang, P. & Yen, C. F. (2002). Posttraumatic stress disorder among adolescent earthquake victims in Taiwan. *Journal of the American Academy of Child and Adolescent Psychiatry, 41,* 875–881.

Jacobs, L. & Wachs, C. (2002). *Parent therapy.* Northvale, NJ: Jason Aronson.

Jalongo, M. R. (1983). Bibliotherapy: Literature to promote socioemotional growth. *Reading Teacher, 36,* 796–803.

Janis, I. L. (1951). *Air war and emotional stress: Psychological studies of bombing and civilian defense.* New York: McGraw-Hill.

Janoff-Bulman, R. (1985). The aftermath of victimization: Rebuilding shattered assumptions. In C. R. Figley (Ed.), *Trauma and its wake* (pp. 15–31). New York: Brunnel/Mazel.

Janoff-Bulman, R. (1992). *Shattered assumptions: Towards a new psychology of trauma.* New York: Free Press.

Johnson, K. (1989). *Trauma in the lives of children: Crisis and stress management techniques for counselors and other professionals.* Alameda, CA: Hunter House.

Johnson, K. (2000). *School crisis management: A hands-on guide to training crisis response team* (2nd ed.). Alameda, CA: Hunter House.

Jones, L. (2000). What are the psychosocial domain and the role of the mental health professional in conflict and post-conflict situations? *Psychosocial Notebook, 1,* 61–70.

Joseph, J. M. (1994). *The resilient child: Preparing today's youth for tomorrow's world.* New York: Plenum Press.

Joseph, S. (1999). Social support and mental health following trauma. In W. Yule (Ed.), *Post-Traumatic stress disorders: Concepts and therapy* (pp. 71–91). New York: Wiley.

Juhnke, G. A. (2002). Intervening with school students after terrorist acts. In D. D. Bass & R. Yep (Eds.), *Terrorism, trauma and tragedies: A counselor's guide for preparing and responding* (pp. 55–58). Alexandria, VA: American Counseling Association.

Kaduson, H. G. & Schaefer, C. E. (Eds.). (2000). *Short-term play therapy for children.* New York: Guilford Press.

Kelly, G. A. (1955). *The psychology of personal constructs.* New York: Norton.

Kenardy, J. A., Webster, R. A., Lewin, T. J., Carr V. J., Hazell, P. L. & Carter, G. L. (1996). Stress debriefing and patterns of recovery following a natural disaster. *Journal of Traumatic Stress, 9,* 37–49.

Kessler, R. C. & McLeod, J. D. (1985). Social support and mental health in community samples. In S. Cohen & S. L. Syme (Eds.), *Social support and health* (pp. 219–240). Orlando, FL: Academic Press.

Kinzie, J. D., Sack, W. H., Angell, R. H. & Manson, S. M. & Rath, B. (1986). The psychiatric effects of massive trauma on Cambodian children. *Journal of the American Academy of Child Psychiatry, 25*, 370–376.

Klingman, A. (1978). Children in stress: Anticipatory guidance in the framework of the educational system. *Personnel and Guidance Journal, 57*, 22–26.

Klingman, A. (1982). Persuasive communication in avoidance behavior: Using role simulation as a strategy. *Simulation and Games, 13*, 37–50.

Klingman, A. (1983). A simulation and simulation games as a strategy for death education. *Death Studies, 7*, 339–352.

Klingman, A. (1985a). Responding to a bereaved classmate: Comparison of two strategies for death education in the classroom. *Death Studies, 9*, 449–454.

Klingman, A. (1985b). Free writing: Evaluation of a preventive program with elementary school children. *Journal of School Psychology, 23*, 167–175.

Klingman, A. (1986). Emotional first aid during the impact phase of a mass disaster. *Emotional First Aid, 3*, 51–57.

Klingman, A. (1987). A school-based emergency crisis intervention in a mass school disaster. *Professional Psychology: Research and Practice, 18*, 205–216.

Klingman, A. (1988). School community in disaster: Planning for intervention. *Journal of Community Psychology, 16*, 205–216.

Klingman, A. (1992). Stress reactions of Israeli youth during the Gulf war: A quantitative study. *Professional Psychology: Research and Practice, 23*, 521–527.

Klingman, A. (1993). School-based intervention following a disaster. In C. F. Saylor (Ed.), *Children and disasters* (pp. 187–210). New York: Plenum Press.

Klingman, A. (1996). School-Based intervention in disaster and trauma. In M. C. Roberts (Ed.), *Model programs in child and family mental health* (pp. 149–171). Mahwah, NJ: Lawrence Erlbaum Associates.

Klingman, A. (2000). Children's affective reactions and coping under threat of uprooting: The case of the Golan Heights. *School Psychology International, 21*, 377–392.

Klingman, A. (2001a). Stress reactions and adaptation of Israeli school-age children evacuated from homes during massive missile attacks. *Anxiety, Stress, and Coping, 14*, 1–14.

Klingman, A. (2001b). Prevention of anxiety disorders: The case of post-traumatic stress disorder. In W. K. Silverman & P. D. A. Treffers (Eds.), *Anxiety disorders in children and adolescents: Research, assessment, and intervention* (pp. 368–391). Cambridge, UK: Cambridge University Press.

Klingman, A. (2002a). Children under war stress. In A. M. La Greca, W. K. Silverman, E. Vernberg & M. C. Roberts (Eds.), *Helping children cope with disasters and terrorism* (pp. 359–380). Washington, DC: American Psychological Association.

Klingman, A. (2002b). School and war. In S. E. Brook, P. J. Lazarus & S. R. Jimerson (Eds.), *Best practices in school crisis prevention and intervention* (pp. 577–598). Bethesda, MD: National Association of School Psychologists.

Klingman, A. (2002c). From supportive-listening to a solution-focused intervention for counselors dealing with political trauma. *British Journal of Guidance and Counselling, 30*, 247–259.

Klingman, A. & Ben-Eli, Z. (1981). A school community in disaster: Primary and secondary prevention in situational crisis. *Professional Psychology: Research and Practice, 12*, 523–533.

Klingman, A. & Hochdorf, Z. (1993). Coping with distress and self harm: The impact of a primary prevention program among eighth grade adolescents. *Journal of Adolescence, 16*, 121–40.

Klingman, A., Koenigsfeld, E. & Markman, D. (1987). Art activity with children following a mass disaster: A preventive crisis intervention modality. *The Arts in Psychotherapy, 14*, 153–166.

Klingman, A. & Kupermintz, H. (1994). Response style and self-control under Scud missile attacks: The sealed room situation during the 1991 Gulf War. *Journal of Traumatic Stress, 7*, 415–426.

Klingman, A., Raviv, A. & Stein, B. (Eds.). (2000). Yeladim bemazavei herum velahatz [Children in stress and emergency situations]. Jerusalem: The Psychological and Counseling Service, Ministry of Education.

Klingman, A., Sagi, A. & Raviv, A. (1993). The effects of war on Israeli children. In L. A. Leavitt & N. A. Fox (Eds.), *Psychological effects of war and violence on children* (pp. 75–92). Hillsdale, NJ: Lawrence Erlbaum Associates.

Klingman, A. & Shalev, R. (2001). Graffiti: The voice of Israeli youth following the assassination of the Prime Minister. *Youth and Society, 32*, 403–420.

Klingman, A., Shalev, R. & Pearlman, A. (2000). Graffiti: A creative means of youth coping with collective trauma. *The Arts in Psychotherapy, 27*, 299–307.

Korol, M., Kramer, T. L., Grace, M. C. & Green, B. L. (2002). Dam break: Long-term follow-up of children exposed to the Buffalo Creek disaster. In A. M. La Greca, W. K. Silverman, E. Vernberg & M. C. Roberts (Eds.), *Helping children cope with disasters and terrorism* (pp. 241–254). Washington, DC: American Psychological Association.

Kostelny, K. & Garbarino, J. (1994). Coping with the consequences of living in danger: The case of Palestinian children and youth. *International Journal of Behavioral Development, 17*, 597–611.

Kronik, A. A., Akhmerov, R. A., Speckhard, A. (1999). Trauma and disaster as life disrupters: A model of computer-assisted psychology applied to adolescent victims of the Chernobyl disaster. *Professional Psychology: Research and Practice, 30*, 586–599.

Kubovi, D. (1982). Therapeutic teaching of literature during the war and it's aftermath. In C. D. Spielberger, I. G. Sarason & A. N. Milgram (Eds.), *Stress and anxiety* (vol. A, pp. 345–349). Washington, DC: Hemisphere.

Kupersmidt, J. B., Shahinfar, A. & Voegler-Lee, E. M. (2002). Children's exposure to community violence. In A. M. La Greca, W. K. Silverman, E. M. Vernberg & M. C. Roberts (Eds.), *Helping children cope with disasters and terrorism* (pp. 381–401). Washington, DC: American Psychological Association.

La Greca, A. M. (2001). Children experiencing disasters. In J. H. Hughes, A. M. La Greca & J. C. Conoley (Eds.), *Handbook of psychological services for children and adolescents* (pp. 195–222). New York: Oxford University Press.

La Greca, A. M. & Prinstien, M. J. (2002). Hurricanes and earthquakes. In A. M. La Greca, W. K. Silverman, E. M. Vernberg & M. C. Roberts (Eds.), *Helping children cope with disasters and terrorism* (pp. 107–138). Washington, DC: American Psychological Association.

La Greca, A. M., Silverman, W. K., Vernberg, E. M. & Roberts, M. C. (Eds.). (2002). *Helping children cope with disasters and terrorism.* Washington, DC: American Psychological Association.

La Greca, A. M., Vernberg, E. M., Silverman, W. K., Vogel, A. & Prinstein, M. J. (1994). *Helping children cope with natural disaster: A manual for school personnel.* Miami, FL: Author.

Lahad, M. (1999). The use of drama therapy with crisis intervention groups, following mass evacuation. *Arts in Psychotherapy, 26*, 27–33.

Lahad, M. & Cohen, A. (1998). Critical incident stress debriefing: The Israeli experience. In O. Ayalon, M. Lahad & A. Cohen (Eds.), *Community stress prevention* (pp. 10–13). Jerusalem: The Psychological and Counseling Service, the Ministry of Education.

Lahad, S., Shacham, Y. & Niv, S. (2000). Coping and community resources in children facing disaster. In A. Y. Shalev, R. Yehuda & A. C. McFarlane (Eds.), *International handbook of human response to trauma* (pp. 389–395). Dordrecht, Netherlands: Kluwer Academic Publishers.

Lahav, R. (1996). What is philosophical counseling? *Journal of Applied Philosophy, 3*, 259–278.

Landau, J., Garrett, J., Shea, R. R., Stanton, D. M., Brikman-Sull, D. & Baceiewicz, G. (2000). Strength in numbers: The ARISE method for mobilizing family and network to engage substance abusers in treatment. *American Journal of Drug and Alcohol Abuse, 26*, 379–398.

Laor, N., Wolmer, L., Mayes, L. C. & Gershon, A. (1997). Israeli preschool children under Scuds: A 30 months follow-up. *Journal of the American Academy of Child and Adolescent Psychiatry, 36*, 349–35.

Laor, N., Wolmer, L., Spirman, S. & Weiner, Z. (2003) Facing war, terrorism, and disaster: Toward a child-oriented comprehensive emergency care system. *Child and Adolescent Psychiatric Clinics of North America, 12*(2), 343–361.

Lavie, P. (2001). Sleep disturbances in the wake of traumatic events. *New England Journal of Medicine, 345,* 1825–1832.

Layne, C. M., Pynoos, R. S., Saltzman, W. R., Arslanagic, B., Black, M., Savjak, N., et al. (2001). Trauma/grief-focused group psychotherapy school-based postwar intervention with traumatized Bosnian adolescents. *Group Dynamics: Theory Research, and Practice, 5,* 277–290.

Lazarus, A. A. (1997). *Brief but comprehensive psychotherapy: The multimodal way.* New York: Springer.

Lazarus, R. S. & Folkman, S. (1984). *Stress, appraisal, and coping.* New York: Springer Verlag.

Ledoux, J. E. & Gorman, J. M. (2001). A call to action: Overcoming anxiety through active coping. *The American Journal of Psychiatry, 158,* 1953–1955.

Lee, J. (2001, October 2). Amid chaos, custodians lend helping hands. *The Spectator: The Stuyvensant High School Newspaper* (New York), p. 7.

Lefcourt, H. M. (2000). The humor solution. In C. R. Snyder (Ed.), *Coping with stress: Effective people and processes* (pp. 68–92). New York: Oxford University Press.

Lefcourt, H. M. & Thomas, S. (1998). Humor and stress revisited. In W. Ruch (Ed.), *The sense of humor: Exploration of a personality characteristic* (pp. 179–202). New York: Mouton de Gruyter.

Lehman, D. (2001, November 10). Substance in Argyle still a mystery. *Glens Falls - Post-Star* (New York), P. 1.

Leonard, A. J. & Burrows, B. (1983). Transition training for high school seniors. *Cognitive Therapy and Research, 7,* 79–92.

Levine, S. (2003, March 24). ERs prepare for another battle front; for hospital worker, the threat is personal. *The Washington Post,* p. B1.

Lichtenstein, R., Schonfeld, D. J., Kline, M. & Speese-Lineham, D. (1995). *How to prepare for and respond to a crisis.* Alexandria, VA: Association for Supervision and Curriculum Development.

Lonigan, C. J., Shannon, M. P., Taylor, C. M., Finch, A. J. & Sall, F. R. (1994). Children exposed to disaster: II. Risk factors for the development of post-traumatic symptomatology. *Journal of the American Academy of Child and Adolescent Psychiatry, 33,* 94–105.

Luthar, S. S. & Zigler, E. (1991). Vulnerability and competence: A review of research on resilience in childhood. *American Journal of Orthopsychiatry, 61,* 6–22.

Mannarino, A. P., Cohen, J. A. & Stubenbort, K. (2002, August). *Treatment of traumatized children after 9/11.* Paper presented at the Child Study Center Grand Rounds Lecture Series, New York University School of Medicine, New York.

March, J. S., Amaya-Jackson L., Murray, M. C., Schulte, A. (1998). Cognitive-behavioral psychotherapy for children and adolescents with posttraumatic stress disorder after a single-incident stressor. *American Academy of Child and Adolescent Psychiatry, 37,* 585–593.

Mash, E. J. & Barkley, R. A. (Eds.). (1998). *Treatment of childhood disorders* (2nd ed.). New York: Guilford Press.

Masten, A. S. & Coatsworth, J. D. (1998). The development of competence in favorable and unfavorable environments: Lessons from research on successful children. *American Psychologist, 53,* 205–220.

Masten, A. S. & Reed, M. G. J. (2002). Resilience in development. In C. R. Snyder & S. J. Lopez (Eds.), *Handbook of positive psychology* (pp. 74–88). London, UK: Oxford University Press.

Mayou, R. A., Ehlers, A. & Hobbs, M. (2000). Psychological debriefing for road traffic accident victims: Three-year follow-up of a randomized controlled trial. *British Journal of Psychiatry, 176,* 589–593.

McCann, I. & Pearlman, L. (1990). Vicarious traumatization: A framework for understanding the psychological effects of working with victims. *Journal of Traumatic Stress, 3,* 131–149.

McFarlane, A. C. (1992). Posttraumatic stress disorder among injured survivors of a terrorist attack: Predictive value of early intrusion and avoidance symptoms. *Journal of Nervous and Mental Disease, 180,* 599–600.

Meichenbaum, D. & Cameron, R. (1983). Stress inoculation training: Toward a general paradigm for training coping skills. In D. Meichenbaum & M. E. Jaremco (Eds.), *Stress inoculation and prevention* (pp. 115–154). New York: Plenum Press.

Merlone, L. & Green, C. (2001). Integrating grief work and therapeutic riding for elementary school students. *School Social Work, 26,* 41–49.

Merrell, K. W. (2001). *Helping students overcome depression and anxiety.* New York: Guilford Press.

Milgram, N. A. & Toubiana, Y. H. (1996). Children's selective coping after a bus disaster: Confronting behavior and perceived support. *Journal of Traumatic Stress, 9,* 687–702.

Milgram, N. A., Toubiana, Y. H., Klingman, A., Raviv, A. & Goldstein, I. (1988). Situational exposure and personal loss in children's acute and chronic stress reactions to a school bus disaster. *Journal of Traumatic Stress, 1,* 339–352.

Miller, G. A. (1969). Psychology as a means of promoting human welfare. *American Psychologist, 24,* 1063–1075.

Minuchin, P. (1985). Families and individual development: Provocations from the field of family therapy. *Child Development, 56,* 289–302.

Mitchell, J. T. (1983). When disaster strikes: The critical incident stress debriefing process. *Journal of the Emergency Medical Services, 8,* 38–43.

Mitchell, J. T. & Everly, G. S. (1997). *Critical incident stress debriefing: An operational manual for the prevention of traumatic stress among emergency services and disaster workers* (2nd ed.). Ellicott City, MD: Chevron.

Moos, R. H. (2002). The mystery of human context and coping: An unrevealing of clues. *American Journal of Community Psychology, 30,* 67–88.

Morrison, J. A., (2000). Protective factors associated with children's emotional responses to chronic community violence exposure. *Trauma, Violence, and Abuse: A Rreview Journal, 1,* 299–320.

Mrazek, P. J. & Haggerty, R. J. (Eds.). (1994). *Reducing risks for mental disorder: Frontiers for preventive intervention research.* Washington, DC: National Academy Press.

Myers, D. (2001). *Weapons of mass destruction and terrorism: Mental health consequences and implications for planning and training.* Paper presented at the Weapons of Mass Destruction/Terrorism Orientation Pilot Program, Clara Barton Center for Domestic Preparedness, Pine Bluff, Arkansas, August, 15–17.

Nader, K. O. (1997). Childhood traumatic loss: The interaction of trauma and grief. In C. R. Figley, B. E. Bride & N. Mazza (Eds.), *Death and trauma: The traumatology of grieving* (pp. 17–39). Washington, DC: Taylor & Francis.

Nader, K. O. (2001). *Terrorism: September 11, 2001 trauma, grief, and recovery.* Retrieved November10, 2002 from http://www.sourcemain.com/gift/Htm/firstaid.htm.

Nader, K. O. (2002). Treating children after violence in schools and communities. In N. B. Webb (Ed.), *Helping Bereaved Children* (pp. 214–244). New York: Guilford Press.

Nader, K. O., Kriegler, J. A., Blake, D. D., Pynoos, R. S., Newman, E. & Weathers F. W. (1996). *Clinician Administered PTSD Scale for Children and Adolescents for DSM-IV (CAPS-CA).* Los Angeles, CA: National Center for PTSD and UCLA Trauma Psychiatry Program, Department of Psychiatry, UCLA School of Medicine.

Nader, K. O. & Mello, C. (2002). Shootings, hostages taking, and children. In A. M. La Greca, W. K. Silverman, E. M. Vernberg & M. C. Roberts (Eds.), *Helping children cope with disasters and terrorism* (pp. 301–326). Washington, DC: American Psychological Association.

Nader, K. O. & Muni, P. (2002). Individual crisis intervention. In S. E. Brock, P. J. Lazarus & S. R. Jimerson (Eds.), *Best practices in school crisis prevention and intervention* (pp. 405–428). Bethesda, MD: National Association of School Psychologists.

Nader, K. O. & Pynoos, R. S. (1991). Play and drawing techniques as tools for interviewing traumatized children. In C. E. Schaffer, K. Gitlin & A. Sandgrund (Eds.), *Play diagnosis and assessment* (pp. 375–389). New York: Wiley.

Nader, K. O. & Pynoos, R. S. (1993). School disaster planning for interventions. *Journal of Social Behavior and Personality, 8,* 299–320.

Nadler, A. (1990). Help-Seeking behavior as a coping resource. In M. Rosenbaum (Ed.), *Learned resourcefulness: On coping skills, self-control, and adaptive behavior* (pp. 128–162). New York: Springer.

National Association of School Psychologists. (2003). *Coping with crisis- Helping children with special needs.* Retrieved September 23, 2003, from http://www.nasponline.org/NEAT/specpop_gen eral.html

National Center for Educational Statistics. (1998). *Violence and discipline problems in U. S. public schools: 1996–97.* Retrieved July 20, 2003, from tttp://www.nces.ed.gov/pubsearch/pubsinfo .asp?pubid=98030

National Institute of Mental Health. (n.d.). *Helping children and adolescents cope with violence and disasters.* Retrieved July 3, 2003, from http://www.nimh.nih.gov/publicat/violence.cfm

Nebbe, L. (2000). Nature therapy. In A. H. Fine (Ed.), *Handbook on animal-assisted therapy: Theoretical foundations and guidelines for practice* (pp. 385–414). San Diago, CA: Academic Press.

Neimeyer, R. A., Keesee, N. J. & Fortner, B. V. (2000). Loss and meaning reconstruction: Propositions and procedures. In R. Malkinson, S. S. Rubin & E. Witztum (Eds.), *Traumatic and nontraumatic loss and bereavement: Clinical theory and practice* (pp. 197–230). Madison, CT: Psychological Press.

Newgass, S. & Schonfeld, D. J. (2000). School crisis intervention, crisis prevention and crisis response. In A. Roberts (Ed.), *Crisis intervention handbook: Assessment, treatment, and research* (2nd ed., pp. 209–228). New York: Oxford University Press.

Newman, M., Black, D. & Harris-Hendriks, J. (1997). Victims of disaster, war, violence, or homicide: Psychological effects on siblings. *Child Psychology and Psychiatry Review, 2,* 140–149.

Nichols, M. P. & Schwartz, R. L. (1998). *Family therapy: Concepts and methods* (4th ed.). New York: Allyn & Bacon.

Niederhoffer, K. G. & Pennebaker, J. W. (2002). Sharing one's story: On the benefits of writing or talking about emotional experience. In C. R. Snyder & S. J. Lopez (Eds.), *Handbook of positive psychology* (pp. 573–583). New York: Oxford University Press.

Noppe, L. D. & Noppe, I. C. (1996). Ambiguity in adolescent understanding of death. In C. A. Corr & D. E. Balk (Eds.), *Handbook of adolescent death and bereavement* (pp. 25–41). New York: Springer.

Norris, F. H., Friedman, M. J., Watson, P. J., Byrne, C. M., Diaz, E. & Kaniasty, K. (2002a). 60,000 disaster victims speak: Part I. An empirical review of the empirical literature, 1981–2001. *Psychiatry, 65*(3), 207–239.

Norris, F. H., Friedman, M. J., Watson, P. J., Byrne, C. M., Diaz, E. & Kaniasty, K. (2002b). 60,000 disaster victims speak: Part II. Summary and implications of the disaster mental health research. *Psychiatry, 65*(3), 240–260.

NYC Board of Education. (2002, May). *Effects of the world trade center attack on New York City public school students.* Retrieved May 5, 2002, from http://nycenet.edu/offices/spss/wtc_needs/cop ing.htm.

Oaklander, V. (2000). Short-term gestalt play therapy for grieving children. In H. G. Kaduson & C. E. Schaefer (Eds.), *Short-term play therapy for children* (pp. 28–52). New York: Guilford Press.

O'Hara, D. M., Taylor, R. & Simpson, K. (1994). Critical incident stress debriefing: Bereavement support in schools: Developing a role for an NLEA educational psychology service. *AEP- Association of Educational Psychologists Journal, 10,* 27–33.

Olson, D. (1997). Family stress and coping: A multisystem perspective. In S. Dreman (Ed.), *The family on the threshold of the 21st century* (pp. 259–280). London: Lawrence Erlbaum.

Omer, H. & Alon, N. (1994). The continuity principle: A unified approach to disaster and trauma. *American Journal of Community Psychology, 22,* 273–285.

Ophir, M. (1980). Mischak hadmaia keshitat tipul becharadah matzavit [Simulation game as an intervention to reduce state anxiety]. In A. Raviv, A. Klingman & M. Horowitz (Eds.), *Yeladim bematzavey lachatz vemashber* (pp. 274–279). Tel Aviv, Israel: Otzar Hamoreh.

Osofsky, J. D. & Scheeringa, M. S. (1997). Community and domestic violence exposure: Effects on development and psychopathology. In D. Cicchetti & S. L. Toth (Eds.), *Rochester Symposium on Developmental Psychopathology: Vol. 8. Developmental perspectives on trauma: Theory, research, and intervention* (pp. 155–180). Rochester, NY: University of Rochester Press.

Pai, M. N. (1969). *Searchlight on sleep disorder.* London: Literary Services and Production.

Pardeck, J. T. & Pardeck, J. A. (1984). Treating abused children through bibliotherapy. *Early Child Development and Care, 16,* 195–203.

Pardess, E. (2002a). *Stories waiting to be told: Children coping with death of a family member express themselves through art in Selah healing retreats.* Tel Aviv, Israel: Crisis Management Center (ICMC/SELAH).

Pardess, E. (2002b). *Support program for bereaved families in the aftermath of tragedy.* Tel Aviv, Israel: Crisis Management Center (ICMC/SELAH).

Pargament, K. I., Cole, B., Vandecreek, L., Belavich, T., Brant, C. & Perez, L. (1999). The vigil: Religion and the search for control in the hospital waiting room. *Journal of Health Psychology, 4,* 327–341.

Parkes, C. M. (1996). *Bereavement: Studies of grief in adult life* (3rd ed.). New York: International University Press.

Pat-Horenczyk, R., Abramovitz, R., Brom, D., Horwitz, S., Baum, N. & Chemtob, C. (2003, October). *Symptoms of PTSD and functional impairment among adolescents exposed to ongoing terror: A comparison between two Israeli contexts.* Paper presented at the meeting of the International Society for Traumatic Stress Studies, Chicago.

Pennebaker, J. W. (1997). Writing about emotional experiences as a therapeutic process. *Psychological Science, 8,* 162–166.

Pennebaker, J. W., Colder, M. & Sharp, L. K. (1990). Accelerating the coping process. *Journal of Personality and Social Psychology, 58,* 528–537.

Perrin, S., Smith, P. & Yule, W. (2000). Practitioner's review: The assessment and treatment of post-traumatic stress disorder in children and adolescents. *Journal of Child Psychology and Psychiatry and Allied Disciplines, 41,* 277–289.

Peterson, C. & Seligman, M. (2003). Character strengths before and after September 11. *Psychological Science, 14,* 381–385.

Pfefferbaum, B. (1997). Posttraumatic stress disorder in children: A review of the past 10 years. *Journal of the American Academy of Psychiatry, 36,* 1503–1511.

Pfefferbaum, B., Nixon, S., Tivis, R., Doughty, D., Pynoos, R. S., Gurwitch, R. H., et al. (2001). Television exposure in children after a terrorist incident. *Psychiatry, 64,* 202–211.

Pfefferbaum, B., Nixon, S., Tucker, P., Tivis, R., Moore, V., Gurevitch, R., et al. (1999). Posttraumatic stress responses in bereaved children after the Oklahoma City bombing. *Journal of the Academy of Child and Adolescent Psychiatry, 38,* 1732–1739.

Pfefferbaum, B., Seale, T., McDonald, N., Brandt, E., Rainwater, S., Maynard, B., et al. (2000). Posttraumatic stress two years after the Oklahoma City bombing in youth geographically distant from the explosion. *Psychiatry, 63,* 358–370.

Pfohl, W. J., Jimerson, S. R. & Lazarus, P. J. (2002). Developmental aspects of psychological trauma and grief. In S. E. Brock, P. J. Lazarus & S. R. Jimerson (Eds.), *Best practices in school crisis prevention and intervention* (pp. 309–353). Bethesda, MD: National Association of School Psychologists.

Phelps, L. F., McCart, M. R. & Davies, W. H. (2002). The impact of community violence on children and parents: Development of contextual assessments. *Trauma, Violence and Abuse, 3* (3), 194–209.

Phillips, T. (2000). Cognitive-behavioral therapy for post-traumatic stress disorder in children and adolescents. In K. N. Dwivedi (Ed.), *Post-traumatic stress disorder in children and adolescents* (pp. 147–162). London: Whurr.

Pitcher, G. & Poland, S. (1992). *Crisis intervention in the schools.* New York: Guilford Press.

Poland, S. (1994). The role of school crisis intervention teams to prevent and reduce school violence and trauma. *School Psychology Review, 23,* 175–189.

Prasad, K. (2000). Biological basis of post-traumatic stress disorder. In K. N. Dwivedi (Ed.), *Post-traumatic stress disorder in children and adolescents* (pp. 39–77). London: Whurr.

Prigerson, H. G., Shear, M. K., Frank, E., Beevy, L. C., Silverman, R., Prigerson, J. et al. (1997). Traumatic grief: A case of loss-induced trauma. *American Journal of Psychiatry, 154,* 1003–1009.

Prinstein, M., La Greca, A. M., Vernberg, E. M., Silverman, W. K. (1996). Children's coping assistance: How parents, teachers, and friends help children cope after a natural disaster. *Journal of Clinical Child Psychology, 25,* 463–475.

Punamaki, R. L. (1996). Can ideological commitment protect children's psychological well-being in situations of political violence. *Child Development, 67,* 55–69.

Punamaki, R. L., Qouta, S. & El Sarraj, E. (1997). Models of traumatic experiences and children's psychological adjustment: The roles of perceived parenting and the children's own resources and activity. *Child Development, 64,* 718–728.

Purvis, J. R., Porter, R. L., Authement, C. C. & Boren, L. C. (1991). Crisis intervention teams in the schools. *Psychology in the schools, 28,* 331–339.

Pynoos, R. S. (1990). Post-traumatic stress disorder in children and adolescents. In B. D. Garfinkle, G. A. Carlson & E. B. Weller (Eds.), *Psychiatric disorder in children and adolescents* (pp. 48–63). Philadelphia: W. B. Saunders.

Pynoos, R. S. & Nader, K. O. (1988). Psychological first aid and treatment approach to children exposed to community violence: Research implications. *Journal of Traumatic Stress, 1,* 445–473.

Pynoos, R. S. & Nader, K. O. (1989). Children's memory and proximity to violence. *Journal of the American Academy of child and adolescent Psychiatry, 28,* 236–241.

Pynoos, R. S., Nader, K. O., Frederick, C., Gonda, L. & Stuper, O. (1987). Grief reactions in school age children following a sniper attack at school. *Israel Journal of Psychiatry and Related Sciences, 24,* 53–63.

Pynoos, R. S., Steinberg, A. M. & Goenjian, A. (1996). Traumatic stress in childhood and adolescence: Recent developments and current controversies. In B. A. van der Kolk, A. C. McFarlane & L. Weisaeth (Eds.), *Traumatic stress* (pp. 331–358). New York: Guilford Press.

Rabalais, A. E., Ruggiero, K. J. & Scotti, J. R. (2002). Multicultural issues in the response of children to disasters. In A. M. La Greca, W. K. Silverman, E. M. Vernberg & M. C. Roberts (Eds.), *Helping child cope with disasters and terrorism* (pp. 73–99). Washington, DC: American Psychological Association.

Rachman, S. J. (1990). *Fear and courage.* New York: W. H. Freeman.

Rando, T. A. (1993). *Treatment of complicated mourning.* Champaign, IL: Research Press.

Raphael, B. (1983). *The anatomy of bereavement.* New York: Basic Books.

Raphael, B. (1997). The interaction of trauma and grief. In D. Black, M. Newman, J. Harris-Hendricks & G. Mezey (Eds.), *Psychological Trauma: A developmental Approach* (pp. 31–43). London: Gaskell/Royal College of Psychiatrists.

Raphael, B., Middleton, W., Martinic, N. O. & Misso, V. (1993). Counseling and therapy of the bereaved. In M. Stroebe, W. Stroebe & R. O. Hansson (Eds.), *Handbook of bereavement: Theory, research and intervention* (pp. 44–61). Cambridge, UK: Cambridge University Press.

Raviv, A. (1993). The use of hotline and media interventions in Israel during the Gulf War. In L. A. Leavitt & N. A. Fox (Eds.), *The psychological effects of war and violence on children* (pp. 319–337). Hillsdale, NJ: Lawrence Erlbaum.

Raviv, A., Sadeh, A., Raviv, A. & Silverstein, O. (1998). The reaction of youth in Israel to the assassination of Prime Minister Yitzhak Rabin. *Political Psychology, 19,* 255–278.

Raviv, A., Sadeh, A., Raviv, A., Silverstein, O. & Diver, O. (2000). Youth Israeli's reactions to national trauma: The Rabin assassination and terror attacks. *Political Psychology, 21,* 299–321.

Realmuto, G. M., Masten, A., Carole, L. F. & Hubbard, J. (1992). Adolescent survivors of massive childhood trauma in Cambodia: Life events and current symptoms. *Journal of Traumatic Stress, 5,* 589–599.

Reilly, I. (2002). Trauma and family therapy: Reflections on September 11 from Northern Ireland. *Journal of Systemic Therapies, 21,* 71–80.

Roberts, D. A. (2001). Religious education as an aid in crisis intervention. In R. G. Stevenson (Ed.), *What will we do? Preparing a school community to cope with crisis* (pp. 60–90). Amityville, NY: Baywood.

Ronen T. (1996). Constructivist therapy with traumatized children. *Journal of Constructivist Psychology, 9,* 139–156.

Ronen, T. (2002). Difficulties in assessing traumatic reactions in children. *Journal of Loss and Trauma, 7,* 87–106.

Rosenblat, P. C. (1993). Grief: The social context of private feelings. In M. S. Stroebe & R. O.

Hansson (Eds.), *Handbook of bereavement: Theory, research, and intervention* (pp. 102–112). Cambridge, UK: Cambridge University Press.

Rotem, T. (2002, September 17). Eizeh min ben adam hy haitah, ilmalay hapiguah. [What kind of person would you have been if it were not for the "hit"]. *Haaretz*, pp. B2-B4.

Rubin, R. H. (1978). Matriarchal themes in black family literature: Implications for family life education. *Family Coordinator, 27*, 33–41.

Rubin, S. S., Malkinson, R. & witztum, E. (2000). Loss, bereavement, and trauma: An overview. In R. Malkinson, S. S. Rubin & E. Witztum (Eds.), *Traumatic and nontraumatic loss and bereavement: Clinical theory and practice* (pp. 5–40). Madison, CT: Psychological Press.

Ryan, V. & Needham, C. (2001). Non directive play therapy with children experiencing psychic trauma. *Clinical Child Psychology and Psychiatry, 6*, 437–453.

Sagi, S. (1998). Effects of personal, family and community characteristics of emotional reactions in stress situation: The Golan Heights negotiations. *Youth and Society, 29*, 311–329.

Saigh, P. A., Green, B. L. & Korol, A. (1996). The history and prevalence of posttraumatic stress disorder with special reference to children and adolescents. *Journal of School Psychology, 34*, 107–131.

Saigh, P. A, Yasik, A. E., Oberfield, R. A., Green, B. L., Halamandaris, P. V., Rubenstein, H., et al. (2000). The children''s PTSD Inventory: Development and reliability. *Journal of Traumatic Stress, 13*, 369–380.

Saigh, P. A., Yule, W. & Inamdar, S. C. (1996). Imaginal flooding of traumatized children and adolescents. *Journal of School Psychology, 34*,163–183

Salmon, K. & Bryant, R. A. (2002). Posttraumatic stress disorder in children: The influence of developmental factors. *Clinical Psychology Review, 22*, 163–188.

Saltzman, W. R., Pynoos, R. S., Layne, C. M., Steinberg, A. M. & Aisenberg, E. (2001). School-based trauma/grief focused group psychotherapy program for youth exposed to community violence. *Group Dynamics, 5*, 291–303.

Saltzman, W. R., Steinberg, A. M., Layne, C. M., Aisenberg, E. & Pynoos, R. S. (2002). A developmental approach to school-based treatment of adolescents exposed to trauma and traumatic loss. *Journal of Child and Adolescent Group Therapy, 11*, 43–56.

Salzer, M. S. & Bickman, L. (1999). The short- and long-term psychological impact of disasters: Implications for mental health interventions and policy. In R. Gist & B. Lubin (Eds.), *Response to disaster: Psychological, community, and ecological approaches* (pp. 63–82). Philadelphia: Brunner/Mazel.

Sande, E. (1998). *Constructing death: The sociology of dying and bereavement.* Cambridge, UK: Cambridge University Press.

Sandoval, J. & Lewis, S. (2002). Cultural considerations in crisis intervention. In S. E. Brock, P. J. Lazarus & S. R. Jimerson (Eds.), *Best practices in school crisis prevention and intervention* (pp. 293–308). Bethesda, MD: National Association of School Psychologists.

Sank, L. I. (1979). Community disasters: Primary prevention and treatment in a health maintenance organization. *American Psychologist, 34*, 334–338.

Sarason, I. G., Sarason, B. R. & Pierce, G. R. (1995). Stress and social support. In S. E. Hobfoll & M. W. De Vries (Eds.), *Extreme stress and communities: Impact and intervention* (pp. 179–197). Dordrecht, Netherlands: Kluwer Academic Publishers.

Sattler, D. N. (2003). Resiliency, posttraumatic growth, and psychological distress after the attacks on America. In *Natural Hazards Research and Applications Information Center, Public Entity Risk Institute, and Institute for Civil Infrastructure Systems, Beyond September 11th: An account of post-disaster research* (pp. 315–332). Special Publication No. 39. Boulder, CO: Natural Hazards Research and Applications Information Center, University of Colorado.

Saylor, C. F. (Ed.). (1993). *Children and disasters.* New York: Plenum Press.

Scheeringa, M. S. & Zeanah, C. H. (2001). A relational perspective on PTSD in early childhood. *Journal of Traumatic Stress, 14*, 799–815.

Scheeringa, M. S., Zeanah, C. H., Drell, M. J. & Larrieu, J. A. (1995). Two approaches to the diagnosis of posttraumatic stress disorder in infancy and early childhood. *Journal of the American Academy of Child and Adolescent Psychiatry, 34*, 191–200.

Schonfeld, D. J. (1993). Talking with children about death. *Journal of Pediatric Health Care, 7*, 269–274.

Schore, A. N. (2001). The effects of early relational trauma on right brain development, affect regulation, and infant mental health. *Infant Mental Health Journal, 22*(1–2), 201–269.

Schwarzwald, J., Weisenberg, M., Waysman, M., Solomon, Z. & Klingman, A. (1993). Stress reactions of school-age children to the bombardment by Scud missiles. *Journal of Abnormal Psychology, 102*, 404–410.

Scott, M. J. (1998). Counseling for trauma and post-traumatic stress disorder. In S. Palmer & G. McMahon (Eds.), *Handbook of counselling* (2nd ed., pp. 473–486). London, UK: Tavistock/Routlage.

Selekman, M. D. (1997). *Solution-focused therapy with children*. New York: Guilford Press.

Seligman, M. E. P. (2002). Positive psychology, positive prevention, and positive therapy. In C. R. Snyder & S. J. Lopez (Eds.), *Handbook of positive psychology* (pp. 3–9). London, UK: Oxford University Press.

Seligman, M. E. P., Reivich, K. J., Jaycox, L. H. & Gillham, J. (1995). *The optimistic child*. New York: Houghton-Mifflin.

Selye, H. (1956). *The stress of life*. New York: McGraw-Hill.

Shahinfar, A. & Fox, N. A. (1997). The effects of trauma on children: Conceptual and methodological issues. In D. Cicchetti & S. L. Toth (Eds.), *Rochester Symposium on Developmental Psychopathology: Vol. 8. Developmental perspectives on trauma: Theory, research, and intervention* (pp. 115–139). Rochester, NY: University of Rochester Press.

Shalev, A. Y. (2002). Acute stress reactions in adults. *Biological Psychiatry, 51*, 532–543.

Shalif, Y. & Leibler, M. (2002). Working with people experiencing terrorist attacks in Israel: A narrative perspective. *Journal of Systemic Therapies, 21*(3), 60–70.

Shapiro, F. (1995). *Eye movement desensitization and reprocessing: Basic principles, protocols and procedures*. New York: Guilford Press.

Shepherd, J. (1990). Victims of personal violence: The relevance of Symondds' model of psychological response and loss-theory. *British Journal of Social Work, 20*, 309–332.

Shepperd, R. (2000). Individual treatments for children and adolescents with post-traumatic stress disorder: Unlocking children's trauma. In K. N. Dwivedi (Ed.), *Post-traumatic stress disorder in children and adolescents* (pp. 131–146). London: Whurr.

Silverman, P. R. (2000). Children as part of the family drama: An integrated view of childhood bereavement. In R. Malkinson, S. S. Rubin & E. Witztum (Eds.), *Traumatic and nontraumatic loss and bereavement: Clinical theory and practice* (pp. 67–90). Madison, CT: Psychological Press.

Silverman, W. K. & La Greca, A. M. (2002). Children experiencing disaster: Definitions, reactions, and predictors of outcome. In A. M. La Greca, W. K. Silverman, E. M., Vernberg & M. C. Roberts (Eds.), *Helping children cope with disaster and terrorism* (pp. 11–33). Washington, DC: American Psychological Association.

Slaikeu, K. A. (1984). *Crisis intervention: A handbook for practice and research*. Boston: Allyn & Bacon.

Solomon, Z. (1988). The effect of combat-related posttraumatic stress disorder on the family. *Journal for the Study of Interpersonal Processes. 51*, 323–329

Solomon, Z. (1995). *Coping with war induced stress: The Gulf War and the Israeli response*. New York: Plenum Press.

Stallard, P. (2000). Debriefing adolescents after critical life events. In B. Raphael & J. P. Wilson (Eds.), *Psychological debriefing: Theory, practice and evidence* (pp. 213–224). New York: Cambridge University Press.

Stamm, B. H. & Friedman, M. J. (2000) Cultural diversity in the appraisal and expression of trauma. In A. Y. Shalev, R. Yehuda & A. C. McFarlane (Eds.), *International handbook of human response to trauma* (pp. 69–85). New York: Kluwer Academic Publishers.

Steinberg, A. (1998). Understanding the secondary traumatic stress of children. In C. R. Figley (Ed.), *Burnout in families: The systematic costs of caring* (pp. 29–46). Boca Raton: CRC Press.

Stern, D. (1995). *The motherhood constellation*. New York: Basic Books.

Stern, M. (2002). *Child-friendly therapy: Biopsychosocial innovations for children and families*. New York: Norton.

Stevenson, E. P. (2002). The school nurse's office: Creating a "Safe Room" in your school. In R. G. Stevenson (Ed.), *What will we do? Preparing a school community to cope with crisis* (pp. 61–68). Amityville, NY: Baywood.

Stewart, A. J., Sokol, M., Healy, J. M. & Chester, N. L. (1986). Longitudinal studies of psychological life change in children and adults. *Journal of Personality and Social Psychology, 61,* 648–658.

Stockes, J. W. & Banderet, L. E. (1997). Psychological aspects of chemical defense and warfare. *Military Psychology, 9,* 395–415.

Stone, B. A. (1998). Self-body-image and PTSD in Australian Spanish speaking trauma survivors. In A. R. Hiscox & A. C. Calish (Eds.), *Tapestry of cultural issues in art therapy* (pp. 176–198). London: Jessica Kingsley.

Sweeney, D. S. & Skurja, C. (2001). Filial therapy as a cross cultural intervention. *Asian Journal of Counseling, 8,* 175–208.

Taylor, R. D. & Wang, M. C. (Eds.). (2000). *Resilience across contexts: Family, work, culture, and community.* Mahwah, NJ: Lawrence Erlbaum Associates.

Taylor, S. E., Klein, L. C., Lewis, B. P., Gruenewald, T. L., Gurung, R. A. R. & Updegraff, J. A. (2000). Biobehavioral responses to stress in females: Tend- and-befriend, not fight-or-flight. *Psychological Review, 103,* 411–429.

Tedeschi, R. G. & Calhoun, L. G. (1995). *Trauma and transformation: Growing in the aftermath of suffering.* Thousand Oaks, CA: Sage.

Tennen, H. & Affleck, G. (2002). Benefit finding and benefit reminding. In C. R. Snyder & S. J. Lopez (Eds.), *Handbook of positive psychology* (pp. 584–579). New York: Oxford University Press.

Terr, L. C. (1983). *Play Therapy.* New York: Wiley Interscience

Terr, L. C. (1985) Children traumatized in small groups. In S. Eth & R. S. Pynoos (Eds.), *Post traumatic stress disorder in children.* Washington, D. C.: American Psychiatric Press.

Terr, L. C. (1989). Treating psychic trauma in children: A preliminary discussion. *Journal of Traumatic Stress, 2,* 2–20.

Terr, L. C. (1990). *Too scared to cry.* New York: Basic Books.

Terr, L. C., Bloch, D. A., Michel,B. A., Shi, H., Reinhardt, J. A. & Metayer, S. (1999). Children's symptoms in the wake of Challenger: A field study of distant-traumatic effects and an outline of related conditions. *American Journal of Psychiatry, 156,* 1536–1544.

Toubiana, Y. H., Milgram, N. A., Strich, Y. & Edelstein, A. (1988). Crisis intervention in a school community disaster: Principles and practices. *Journal of Community Psychology, 16,* 228–240.

Trappler, B. & Friedman, S. (1996). Posttraumatic stress disorder in survivors of the Brooklyn Bridge shooting. *American Journal of Psychiatry, 153,* 705–707.

Trump, K. S. (2000). *Classroom killers? Hallways hostages? How school can prevent and manage school crisis.* Thousand Oaks, CA: Corwin Press.

Ulrich, R. S. (1993). Biophilia, biophobia, and natural landscapes. In S. R. Kellert & E. O. Wilson (Eds.), *The biophilia hypothesis* (pp. 73–137). Washington, DC: Island Press/Shearwater Books.

van der Kolk, B. A. (1997). The complexity of adaptation to trauma: Self-regulation, stimulation, discrimination, and characterological development. In B. A. van der kolk, A. C. McFarlane & L. Weisaeth (Eds.), *Traumatic stress* (pp. 43–182). New York: Guilford Press.

van der Kolk, B. A. & Fisler, R. (1995). Dissociation and the fragmentary nature of traumatic memories: Overview and exploratory study. *Journal of Traumatic Stress, 8,* 505–525.

van der Kolk, B. A., McFarlane, A. C. & Weiseth, L. (1996). *Traumatic Stress.* New York: Guilford Press.

Verlinden, S., Hersen, M. & Thomas, J. (2000). Risk factors in school shootings. *Clinical Psychology Review, 20,* 3–56.

Vernberg, E. M. (1999). Children's response to disasters: Family and system approaches. In R. Gist & B. Lubin (Eds.), *Response to disaster: Psychosocial, community, and ecological approaches* (pp. 193–209). Philadelphia: Brunner/Mazel.

Vernberg, E. M. (2002). Intervention approaches following disaster. In A. M. La Greca, W. K. Silverman, E. M. Vernberg & M. C. Roberts (Eds.), *Helping children cope with disasters and terrorism* (pp. 55–72). Washington, DC: American Psychological Association.

Vernberg, E. M., La Greca, A. M., Silverman, W. K. & Prinstein, M. J. (1996). Predictors of children's post-disaster functioning following Hurricane Andrew. *Journal of Abnormal Psychology, 105*, 237–248.

Vernberg, E. M. & Varela, R. E. (2001). Posttraumatic stress disorder: A developmental psychopathology of anxiety. In M. W. Vasey & M. R. Dadds (Eds.), *The developmental psychopathology of anxiety* (pp. 386–406). New York: Oxford University Press.

Watts, R. E. & Broaddus, J. L. (2002). Improving parent-child relationships through filial therapy: An interview with Garry Landreth. *Journal of Counseling and Development, 80*, 272–279.

Webb, N. B. (Ed.). (1991). *Play therapy with children in crisis.* New York: Guilford Press.

Webb, N. B. (2002a). The child and death. In N. B., Webb (Ed.), *Helping Bereaved Children* (pp. 3–18). New York: Guilford Press.

Webb, N. B. (2002b). Counseling and therapy for the bereaved child. In N. B., Webb (Ed.), *Helping Bereaved Children* (pp. 247–264). New York: Guilford Press.

Weisaeth, L. (1995). Preventive psychological interventions after disaster. In S. E. Hobfoll & M. W. De Vries (Eds.), *Extreme stress and communities: Impact and intervention* (pp. 401–419). Dordrecht, Netherlands: Kluwer Academic Publishers.

Weisenberg, M., Schwarzwald, J., Waysman, M., Solomon, Z. & Klingman, A. (1993). Coping of school-age children in the sealed room during Scud missile bombardment and post-war stress reactions. *Journal of Consulting and Clinical Psychology, 61*, 462–467.

White, M. (2002). *Attending to the consequences of trauma.* Workshop Notes. Retrieved December 22, 2003 from http://dulwichcenter.com.au

White, M. & Epston, D. (1991). *Narrative means to therapeutic ends.* New York: W. W. Norton.

Wolmer, L., Laor, N. & Yazgan, Y. (2003). School reactivation programs after disaster: Could teachers serve as clinical mediators? *Child and Adolescent Psychiatric Clinics of North America, 12* (2), 363–381

Woodcock, J. (2000). Refugee children and their families: Theoretical and clinical perspectives. In K. N. Dwivedi (Ed.), *Post-traumatic stress disorder in children and adolescents (pp. 213–239).* London: Whurr.

Woodruff, C. R. (2002). Pastoral counselling: An American perspective. *British Journal of Guidance and Counselling, 30*, 93–101.

Wright, J. & Chung, M. C. (2001). Mystery or mastery? Therapeutic writing: A review of the literature. *British Journal of Guidance and Counselling, 29*, 277–291.

Wright, M. O., Masten, A. S. & Hubbard, J. J. (1997). Long-term effects of massive trauma: Developmental and psychobiological perspectives. In D. Cicchetti & S. L. Toth (Eds.), *Rochester Symposium on Developmental Psychopathology: Vol. 8. Developmental perspectives on trauma: Theory, research, and intervention*

Yehuda, R. (2002). Post-traumatic stress disorder. *New England Journal of Medicine, 346*, 108–114.

Yule, W. (1992). Post-traumatic stress disorder in child survivors of shipping disasters: The sinking of the "Jupiter". *Psychotherapy and Psychosomatics, 57*, 200–205.

Yule, W. (2001). Post-traumatic stress disorder in children and adolescents. *International Review of Psychiatry, 13*, 194–200.

Yule, W., Perrin, S. & Smith (2000). Traumatic events and post-traumatic stress disorder. In W. K. Silverman & P. D. A. Treffers (Eds.), *Anxiety disorders in children and adolescents: Research, assessment, and intervention* (pp. 212–234). Cambridge, U. K: Cambridge University Press.

Yule, W., Udwin, O. & Bolton, D. (2002). Mass transportation disaster. In A. M. La Greca, W. K. Silverman, E. Vernberg & M. C. Roberts (Eds.), *Helping children cope with disasters and terrorism* (pp. 223–240). Washington, DC: American Psychological Association.

Zeidner, M., Klingman, A., & Itskovitz, R. (1993). Children's reactions and coping under threat of missile attack: A semi-projective assessment procedure. *Journal of Personality Assessment, 60*, 435–457.

Ziv, A. & Israeli, R. (1973). Effects of bombardment on the manifested anxiety level of children living in the Kibbutz. *Journal of Consulting and Clinical Psychology, 40*, 287–291.

Index

Absenteeism
    postdisaster, 124–126
    posttraumatic stress disorder-related, 50
Academic performance, posttraumatic decline
    in, 28, 178
Acute stress disorder, 17, 29, 47
    definition of, 51
    in Israeli adolescents, 78
    as posttraumatic stress disorder risk factor,
        51
Adaptation
    to bereavement, 54
    developmental processes and, 177–178
    effect of family functioning on, 63–68
    effect of family support on, 32
    effect of parents on, 63–68
        implications for interventions, 64–65
        mechanisms of, 65–68
    resiliency as, 79
    to war, 77–78
Adapted Family Debriefing Model, 135
Adolescents
    depression treatment in, 194
    developmental tasks of, 95
    fear of school violence in, 6
    grief processes in, 56
    ideology-related coping in, 30–31
    posttraumatic stress disorder in, 96
    posttraumatic symptomatology in, 29
    risk-taking behavior of, 95–96
    school-based group therapy for, 191–192
    trauma responses in, 95–96
    use of humor by, 142
Adults. *See also* Parents; Teachers
    influence on children's trauma responses,
        94–95

Age factors, in posttraumatic
    symptomatology, 28–29
Aggression
    bereavement-related, 56
    posttraumatic, 28
    posttraumatic stress disorder-related, 50,
        177
Agitated behavior, posttraumatic stress
    disorder-related, 49
Alcohol abuse, bereavement-related, 56
Amnesia, dissociative, 51
Anger
    bereavement-related, 53, 54, 55
    posttraumatic, 46
    posttraumatic stress disorder-related, 49
Anniversaries, of traumatic events, 122, 123,
        180
Anthrax, mailings of, 5, 36
Antisocial behavior, posttraumatic, 29
Anxiety
    habituation of, 186, 192
    over-prediction of, 78
    posttraumatic, 18, 25, 46
    posttraumatic stress disorder-related, 52
    school-based group therapy for, 194
    terrorism-related, 36
Anxiety disorders, screening for, 183
Anxiety management training, 192
Arousal. *See* Hyperarousal
Arts, expressive, 142–144
    use in narrative therapy, 188
    use in nature-assisted interventions, 146–
        147
ASD. *See* Acute stress disorder
Assumptions, effect of traumatic events on,
        48, 148